The Human Becoming
School of Thought

The Lord God formed man out of the clay of the ground and blew into his nostrils the breath of life, and so man became a living being. Gen. 2: 7-9.

The Human Becoming School of Thought

A Perspective for Nurses and Other Health Professionals

Rosemarie Rizzo Parse

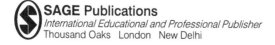

SAGE Publications
International Educational and Professional Publisher
Thousand Oaks   London   New Delhi

The cover art was designed by Alj Mary for the original work *Man-Living-Health: A Theory of Nursing.* The black and white colors represent apparent opposites—paradox—which is signficant to the ontology of human becoming. The green is the color of hope, representing ongoing human-universe emergence. The center joining of the swirling ribbons represents the cocreated mutual human-universe process at the ontological level and the nurse-person process and researcher-participant process at the methodological level. The combination of the green and black swirls intertwining represents human-universe cocreation as an ongoing process of becoming.

For information:

SAGE Publications, Inc.
2455 Teller Road
Thousand Oaks, California 91320
E-mail: order@sagepub.com

SAGE Publications Ltd.
6 Bonhill Street
London EC2A 4PU
United Kingdom

SAGE Publications India Pvt. Ltd.
M-32 Market
Greater Kailash I
New Delhi 110 048 India

Printed in the United States of America

Library of Congress Cataloging-in-Publication Data

Parse, Rosemarie Rizzo.
    The human becoming school of thought: A perspective for nurses and other health professionals / by Rosemarie Rizzo Parse.
    p. cm.
    Rev. ed. of: Man-living-health. c1981.
    Includes bibliographical references and index.
    ISBN 0-7619-0582-0 (cloth : acid-free paper)
    ISBN 0-7619-0583-9 (pbk. : acid-free paper)
    1. Nursing—Philosophy. I. Parse, Rosemarie Rizzo.
Man-living-health. II. Title.
    RT84.5 .P357 1998
    610.73'01—ddc21   98-8893

98 99 00 01 02 03 10 9 8 7 6 5 4 3 2 1

Acquiring Editor:	Dan Ruth
Editorial Assistant:	Anna Howland
Production Editor:	Sherrise M. Purdum
Production Assistant:	Karen Wiley
Typesetter/Designer:	Danielle Dillahunt
Cover Designer:	Ravi Balasuriya
Print Buyer:	Anna Chin

CONTENTS

ACKNOWLEDGMENTS

I acknowledge with appreciation the many predecessors, contemporaries, and successors who continue to coconstitute the evolution of the human becoming school of thought. Special thanks and affection go to those people who lived and participated with the creation of this work and bore witness at many realms of the universe to its birthing.

- John A. Parse, husband and friend, "the wind beneath my wings," whose loving presence, limitless support, and fine-honed writing ability immeasurably aid all of my projects.
- Rosella M. Obringer and Frank J. Rizzo, my insightful, loving parents, their children, and their children's children, whose enlivening presences are always with me.
- April L. Hackathorn, colleague and friend, a gift in my life, whose gentle urgings, calm presence, precise copyediting, and generous assistance are invaluable in my many projects.
- A once and future friend, whose ever present metaperspective on my many emerging projects illuminates the struggles and the moments of joy all-at-once.

PREFACE TO THE 1998 EDITION

This revision was born against the backdrop of a vastly changing global health care scene. These changes alter significantly the substantive nature of disciplinary contributions to the health of society. Nurses, physicians, and other health care providers are restructuring their approaches to people and redefining the boundaries of their disciplines. There is a global move toward more concern for the perspective of the person and family to satisfy the concerns of the public for more humane treatment, yet at the same time there is a growing trend toward diminishing services, with the blurring of disciplinary boundaries and cross-education of health care providers to lower the cost of health care.

The original work was a theory of nursing, but over time, with the development of the research and practice methodologies, it evolved into a school of thought. A school of thought is "a theoretical point of view held by a community of scholars" (Parse, 1997c, p. 74). It is a knowledge tradition, including a specific ontology (assumptions and principles), a specified epistemology (focus of inquiry), and congruent methodologies (approaches to research and practice). The term *theory* refers to the principles of human becoming.

The human becoming school of thought, with its focus on the perspective of the person, family, and community, is particularly important as we approach the 21st century. There is growing interest among nurses worldwide for a theoretical perspective to guide research and practice that centers on the person's, family's, and community's views. Not only nurses but other health care providers are searching for ways to be with others as they enhance their quality of life. Human becoming provides a framework to guide nurses and others in research on lived experiences and in practice that honors personal beliefs about health and quality of life.

Since 1981, the theory has been used widely in research and practice. Three books further elaborating the theory have been published (Parse, 1987, 1995; Parse, Coyne, & Smith, 1985). Many articles and book chapters have also been published, and the community of nurse scholars and others have embraced the work as a viable option to guide nursing research and practice. The theory is now used as a guide to practice in settings in Canada, Finland, Sweden, and the United States, and research projects with the Parse research method are being conducted in Australia, Canada, Denmark, Finland, Greece, Italy, Japan, Korea, Sweden, Taiwan, the United Kingdom, and the United States. Books, chapters, and articles have been translated into many languages.

The original assumptions, principles, and theoretical structures, with their various explanations, are updated here to reflect the current language and any new knowledge. Some additions clarify the position of human becoming as a human science. One completely new chapter has been added to elaborate on the research and practice methodologies because these were constructed after the 1981 book was published.

The book focuses on the human-universe-health process—the phenomenon of concern to the discipline—and is primarily intended for professional nurses and other health care providers, researchers, faculty, and students concerned with quality of life from the perspective of the people they serve. It is for those who value research and practice guided by a nursing theory and those who believe that humans in mutual process with the universe structure meaning multidimensionally, coauthor health, freely choose ways of becoming, and move beyond each moment with hopes and dreams. This second edition is offered in the ongoing quest of defining unique nursing knowledge for the betterment of humankind.

—*Rosemarie Rizzo Parse, RN, PhD, FAAN*

PREFACE TO THE 1981 EDITION

There is an alive and growing force within nursing today generating energy toward the advancement of nursing as a scientific discipline. This book articulates a theory of nursing that supports this growing force.

The intent of this work is to set forth a different paradigm of nursing, a theory rooted in the human sciences, an alternative to the traditional. The different paradigm is the theory of nursing as Man[1]-Living-Health. This theory was genealogically created to enhance nursing's unique body of knowledge. The idea to create such a theory began many years ago when I began to wonder and wander and ask why not? The theory itself, as articulated in this book, surfaced in me in Janusian fashion over the years in interrelationship with others, primarily through my lived experience with nursing. The creation of it has been long and arduous, but with many moments of joy. The components have been seen, at times, as through a glass darkly. They have been elusive, abstract, and disparate—and often, just beyond my reach. To present the theory in this book appears to say "it is finished!" Yet the theory has only just begun to be viewed and enhanced by those who take up the challenge to evolve nursing science to a higher level of complexity and specificity. While the written theory follows in the pages of this book, the nuances and mysteries of it continue to stir in me new ideas, yet different ways of viewing Man-Living-Health. It is hoped the ideas herein will spark different thoughts, shed new lights, and mobilize shifts in points of view.

The work is primarily intended for graduate students at both master's and doctoral levels, as well as for faculty in baccalaureate and higher-degree programs who might find it useful in curriculum development. It is offered as a contribution in the ongoing quest of defining a unique body of nursing knowledge.

Note

1. *Man*, throughout the text, refers to *Homo sapiens*.

—Rosemarie Rizzo Parse, PhD, RN, FAAN

CHAPTER 1

EMERGENCE OF A
NEW PARADIGM OF NURSING

To posit the idea of nursing grounded in the human sciences is to make explicit an alternative to the traditional practice of nursing as a medical model grounded in the natural sciences. Historically, nursing has been a health profession closely related to medicine in the cure of human beings, but it is now justifying its claims as a discipline. Many variables are related to the fact that nursing has held tenaciously to its medical connections and theories. These include the role of women in history and the power of organized medicine. Nursing's close association with medicine has understandably led to its ontological and methodological grounding in the natural sciences. There is a significant difference between a natural science approach and a human science approach. Natural sciences posit methodologies that elicit quantitative data from observable phenomena and reveal causal relationships. Natural sciences deal with the reduction to parts of the phenomena being studied. These parts are examined by using criteria from a predetermined theoretical framework. "The working model of the natural sciences is constituted by the concepts of a causal order in a physical world and their particular methodology consists of procedures for discovering it" (Dilthey, 1961, p. 109).

Philosophically, nursing has adopted the natural science model of the human historically employed by medical science, *Homo naturus*. The major idea underpinning this medical model is a particulate view of the human. Curricula in nursing programs and nursing textbooks are still organized into the classical divisions of medical-surgical, pediatric, obstetric, and psychiatric nursing, paralleling the medical specialties. Though the content is still the same, these divisions are sometimes called by different names, for example, "adult health" for medical-surgical nursing and "maternal-child" for obstetrics and pediatrics. The education and practice of advanced practice nurses follow the medical model path even more closely, since these nurses assume the traditional physician's tasks of diagnosing medical diseases and prescribing medications and other treatments (Parse, 1994a). Research studies in nursing using methodologies studies in nursing using from the physical sciences deal with disease or trauma and the attendant treatment and cure. "Tasks, technology and teaching have been the predominant nursing frames of reference . . . from a reading of the first 25 years of *Nursing Research*" (Ellis, 1977, p. 181), and they still are in the late 1990s. More specifically, natural science nursing has, since its inception, dealt with the quantification of the human and illness rather than the qualification of the human's total health experience. The human has been, and most often still is, approached through the study of parts rather than through the study of unitary patterns. The human's participative experience with health has been virtually ignored.

The most predominant theoretical approach in nursing, then, posits the human as a bio-psycho-socio-spiritual organism, and this approach is in keeping with the natural science medical model view. The medical model, nearly as far back as Galen, has focused on a certain mind-body dichotomy, a Cartesian dualism that predates Descartes by centuries but still permeates much modern thinking. This dualism has been successful in the practice of medicine as medicine, and in the emergence of medical science. To treat *Homo naturus* medically is to deal with biological-physiological-psychosocial systems in which tissues, organs, and their various diseases are viewed and treated separately. Nursing's emergence with medicine in the study of the human created one science, namely, medical science, with the coparticipation of both medicine and nursing. This approach seriously curtailed the development of a unique and distinct body of nursing knowledge, even though Florence Nightingale (1859/1946) set forth a view of the human that could be interpreted as more than the sum of parts, a view of nursing as knowledge distinct from medical knowledge, and a focus on health rather than illness. And, even though Hildegard Peplau in 1952 pioneered nursing as a science by authoring a unique work, *Interpersonal Relations in Nursing*, in the main, nursing, philosophically and in practice, still mirrors the natural science approach and, with only some exceptions, follows the medical model.

Conceptual approaches to nursing, differing slightly from the traditional medical model nursing, emerged over the last three decades. These conceptualizations, although still adhering in part to medical science, incorporate notions of open systems, total and holistic views of the human, adaptation, self-care, caring, and interactional and transactional relations (I. M. King, 1981; Leininger, 1996; Neuman, 1982; Orem, 1995; Paterson & Zderad, 1976; Roy & Andrews, 1991; Watson, 1988). Other scholars (Newman, 1994; Parse, 1981; Rogers, 1970) have created conceptualizations drastically different from the natural science medical model nursing, heralding nursing as a basic science. The emergence of a variety of conceptual systems of nursing bears witness to the coming of age of nursing as a discipline. The discipline of nursing is emerging, as do all disciplines, through a process of formal research and conceptual development, from the prescientific phase to the scientific phase, with different paradigmatic perspectives of the phenomenon of concern. The emergence began with the institution of formal nursing in the middle of the 19th century, when prescientific practice was based on experience under an informal structure. Nursing continues to emerge as a scientific discipline, with the formalized structure embedded in its frameworks and theories.

Although most nurse scholars today agree that nursing is a science with the human-universe-health process as the phenomenon of concern, some believe that it is an *applied* science (drawing knowledge from all other sciences), and others believe that it is a *basic* science with its own body of distinct knowledge. Applied science nursing is the totality paradigm view in which the human is considered a bio-psycho-socio-spiritual being made up of distinct parts: body, mind, and spirit. The definition of health is physical, psychological, social, and spiritual well-being, and the human-universe process is considered adaptive. The totality paradigm is consistent with the medical science perspective, and scholars from this paradigm foster research and practice consistent with natural science tenets (Parse, 1987). Basic science nursing is the simultaneity paradigm view in which the human is considered unitary, an indivisible being recognized through patterns, and the human-universe process is mutual ongoing change. The simultaneity paradigm is a unique nursing perspective, and scholars from this paradigm foster research and practice consistent with human science tenets (Parse, 1987).

The Human Becoming School of Thought is grounded in the human sciences. The work is consistent with Martha E. Rogers' principles and postulates about the human and with major tenets and concepts from existential-phenomenological thought, but it is a new product, a different conceptual system. Rogers (1970) explicitly inaugurated the simultaneity paradigm when she authored the landmark book *An Introduction to the Theoretical Basis of Nursing* and created the first definitive basic nursing science conceptual framework. A conceptual framework represents "a matrix of concepts which together describe the focus of inquiry" (Newman, 1979, pp. 5-6). Rogers' work is rooted in Ludwig von Bertalanffy's general system theory and in the works of Teilhard de Chardin, Michael Polanyi, and Kurt Lewin. Søren Kierkegaard, a nonphenomenologist, founded existentialism; Edmund Husserl, a nonexistentialist, created phenomenology. Kierkegaard and Husserl interface in their view of the human as more than atomistic. Martin Heidegger first recognized the congruence of these two authors' thoughts and merged existentialism and phenomenology to create existential phenomenology. The existential-phenomenological movement, evolved primarily through Heidegger, was promulgated and disseminated widely through the works of Jean-Paul Sartre, Maurice Merleau-Ponty, and others. Rogers, Heidegger, Sartre, and Merleau-Ponty, then, are the predominant theorists drawn on in the creation of the ontology of human becoming. Others included Buber, Marcel, Tillich, van den Berg, and van Kaam. Important literary influences in this endeavor were Camus, Kafka, and Simone de Beauvoir.

To draw upon the works of these scholars, of course, is to build on a solid foundation and to maintain a bridge to the past necessary in the establishment of any scientific work. Earlier in the 20th century and continuing into the present, these various scholars and their works were as much criticized as acclaimed, as much reviled as admired, and as much ignored as followed. Consistent with history dating back to Darwin, Copernicus, and beyond, these plowers of new ground and creators of new views found the initial going difficult. Their problems have been partially of their own making. In *The Structure of Scientific Revolutions*, Thomas S. Kuhn (1970) writes that, in solving a problem or forming a theory, a scientist has two choices. The scientist may attempt to solve the problem within the existing system, as Copernicus could have attempted within the Ptolemaic theory, or the scientist may create a new system, a counterinstance, a revolutionary process. The Darwins, Copernicuses, Kierkegaards, Husserls, and Rogerses of the world have chosen the latter.

To do so, of course, is to wander in the wilderness, to want for honor, and to lack disciples, at least for a time. Ultimately, and happily, the Copernicuses have their Galileos, the Darwins their Huxleys, and the Kierkegaards and Husserls their Heideggers. Rogers, too, has her major disciples, such as Elizabeth A. M. Barrett, Violet Malinski, and John R. Phillips, and she continues to attract more. To follow Rogers, of course, is to forsake the theory of medicine as a paradigm of nursing and to affirm a different conceptual system based on the unitary human being.

A paradigm in any science usually emerges when the scientists of that particular discipline recognize an anomaly between existing theory and the nature of the phenomenon it seeks to describe (Kuhn, 1970). Those scientists who stimulate the change, those visionaries who create the new paradigm, view the anomaly as more than just a puzzle. Puzzles, after all, are the historic and daily challenges, the ones that can ultimately be solved within the existing order. Forward-looking scientists instead view this anomaly as a real counterinstance, a crisis situation, one requiring a new articulation of the relationships among the phenomena and calling for a different view of the fundamentals. Lavoisier, for example, promulgated such a view when he published his theory on chemical compounds, diverging forever from the elemental earth theory of Priestley and others.

Recognition of an anomaly between the theories of medicine and the nature of nursing is at the center of the emergence of the new paradigm for nursing grounded in the human sciences. The theories of medicine and applied science nursing are grounded in the view of the human as a mechanistic bio-psycho-socio-spiritual being, the sum of parts. Consequently, practice focuses on diagnosis and treatment in curing, controlling, and preventing disease. In contrast, the nature of basic science nursing is grounded in the view of the human as unitary (different from the sum of parts) and focuses on optimal well-being (Rogers, 1970, 1992) and quality of life (Parse, 1981, 1992, 1995, 1997a). Thus, basic science nursing has a different root and focus from medicine. This fundamental difference is not viewed as a puzzle to be solved but as a counterinstance of the same type and mode of crisis just described. A crisis of that proportion requires a different fundamental view of the familiar. The nursing paradigm elaborated in this book identifies the unitary human as one who coparticipates with the universe in creating becoming, and who is whole, open, and free to choose ways of becoming. This is in contradistinction to a paradigm that views the human as the sum of parts, acted on and delimited by such forces as disease and pathology.

The emergence of a new paradigm of nursing grounded in the human sciences is illuminated in the description and explanation of the human becoming school of thought in the following chapters. Rogers' three principles—*helicy, complementarity* (in 1986, Rogers renamed this *integrality*), and *resonancy*—as well as the postulates energy field, openness, pattern, and four-dimensionality (Rogers changed this term to *multidimensionality* in 1990 and then *pandimensionality* in 1992) are explained. The fundamental tenets of existential phenomenology, human subjectivity, and intentionality, with the ideas of coconstitution, coexistence, and situated freedom, are also discussed, since the human becoming assumptions are congruent with Rogerian science and tenets from existential phenomenology.

Assumptions about the human and becoming emerge from a synthesis of these principles, postulates, tenets, and concepts. These assumptions are explicated, and the principles, concepts, and theoretical structures of human becoming are explained. The research and practice methodologies of the human becoming school of thought are discussed in detail. A sample of some aspects of a curriculum plan grounded in the human becoming school of thought is proposed for a program leading to a master's of science in nursing degree.

CHAPTER 2

EVOLUTION OF THE HUMAN BECOMING SCHOOL OF THOUGHT

The human becoming school of thought is rooted in the human sciences, which posit methodologies directed toward uncovering the meaning of phenomena as humanly experienced. Human science methodologies are used to study the unitary human's participative experience with a situation. "The human sciences are possible only because we directly participate in their subject matter" (Macquarrie, 1968, p. 36). They aim at understanding the connectedness of life itself (Dilthey, 1961). The methods of inquiry lead to the creation of theoretical structures about the meaning of lived experiences. The notion of human science arose from the works of Wilhelm Dilthey (1833-1911), a German philosopher. Dilthey's concern is that the natural sciences when applied to human living do not capture the meaning of life (Dilthey, 1894/1977a, 1927/1977b; Ermarth, 1978). His focus is on the interconnectedness of humans with the world, and he proposes developing the human sciences to enhance the understanding of experiences as humanly lived. Dilthey believes that the human sciences should illuminate meanings, values, and relationships. Others have forged the path that

Dilthey initiated to bring to light the values and importance of the human sciences (Gadamer, 1976; Giorgi, 1970, 1971, 1985; Heidegger, 1962; Polkinghorne, 1983; Ricoeur, 1974). The ontology of human becoming posited in this book has as a fundamental tenet the unitary human's participation in health; thus, the research and practice methodologies focus on experiences as humanly lived.

The human becoming school of thought is a human science system of interrelated concepts describing the unitary human's mutual process with the universe in cocreating becoming. Essential ideas are the human-universe mutual process, the coconstitution of health, the multidimensional meanings the unitary human gives to being and becoming, and the human's freedom in each situation to choose alternative ways of becoming.

The theory (principles) of human becoming is built on assumptions about humans and becoming congruent with Rogers' principles and postulates and with existential-phenomenological thought, primarily of Heidegger, Sartre, and Merleau-Ponty. Postulates from Rogers' nursing science correspond with von Bertalanffy's general system theory and are synthesized with concepts from existential-phenomenological thought to create the assumptions of human becoming. Table 2.1 is a comparison of the human becoming school of thought, Rogers' science of unitary human beings, and totality paradigm theories.

The next two sections explain the principles and postulates from the science of unitary human beings and the tenets and concepts from existential phenomenology that have been synthesized in the creation of the assumptions of human becoming.

Principles and Postulates of the Science of Unitary Human Beings

Rogers posits three major principles of nursing science—helicy, integrality, and resonancy—and four postulates—energy field, openness, pattern, and pandimensionality. These are the specific ideas from Rogers used in the creation of the assumptions of human becoming.

TABLE 2.1 Comparison of Nursing Paradigms

	Simultaneity		Totality
	Human Becoming	Science of Unitary Human Beings	All Totality Theories
Human being	Open being cocreating meaning in multidimensional mutual process with the universe	Energy field in mutual process with environmental field	Bio-psycho-socio-spiritual organism interacting with environment
	Recognized by patterns of relating	Recognized by field pattern	Recognized by physiological, psychological, sociological, and spiritual attributes
	Freely chooses in situation	Participates knowingly in change	Interacts by coping with or managing the environment
Health	Cocreated process of becoming as experienced and described by the person, family, and community	A value	Physical, psychological, social, and spiritual well-being as defined by norms
Central phenomenon of nursing	Unitary human's becoming	Unitary human beings	Self-care, adaptation, goal attainment, or caring
Goal of the discipline of nursing	Quality of life	Well-being and optimal health	Promotion of health and prevention of disease
Mode of inquiry	Qualitative: Parse's research method; human becoming hermeneutic method	Quantitative and qualitative methods	Extant quantitative and qualitative methods
Mode of practice	True presence in all-at-once illuminating meaning through explicating, synchronizing rhythms through dwelling with, mobilizing transcendence through moving beyond	Pattern manifestation appraisal Pattern profile Perceptions Expressions Experiences Deliberative mutual patterning	Nursing process with nursing diagnoses

Principles

Helicy

The principle of helicy specifies the "continuous, innovative, unpredictable, increasing diversity of human and environmental field patterns" (Rogers, 1992, p. 31). This principle elaborates the nature of change. It relates to the postulates of energy field and pandimensionality.

Integrality

The principle of integrality specifies the "continuous mutual human field and environmental field process" (Rogers, 1992, p. 31). This principle elaborates the continuity in the process of change and relates to the postulates of energy field and openness.

Resonancy

The principle of resonancy specifies the "continuous change from lower to higher frequency wave patterns in human and environmental fields" (Rogers, 1992, p. 31). The rhythmical energy of the human with the environment is expressed in wave patterns specifying the direction of change. This principle relates to the postulates of openness and pattern.

Postulates

Energy Field

Rogers (1970) posits the unitary human as an indivisible energy field. She says that the unity of the human is a reality: The human "is a unified whole possessing . . . integrity and manifesting characteristics that are more than and different from the sum of . . . parts" (p. 47). Humans transcend the deductions made from the study of chemistry, biology, psychology, and sociology and cannot be explained by the ideated integration of parts. This idea of the unitary human dates back to the ancient Greeks; with emergent technologies, more and more emphasis was directed toward the study of the segments of the human. Yet, the human cannot be totalized by an additive process. The human field is in mutual process with the environmental field.

Polanyi (1958) supports the view of the human as more than and different from the sum of parts: "Understanding of a whole appreciates the coherence of its subject matter and thus acknowledges the existence of a value that is absent from the constituent particular" (p. 327). To study unitary humans, then, means to study human wholeness, the characteristics of which emerge through pattern. The energy field is infinite, in continuous motion, and the fundamental unit of the living and nonliving (Rogers, 1992).

Openness

This postulate refers to the human as an open system, an energy field contiguous with the environment. Rogers (1970) negates the human as a closed system, a steady state, and an adaptive organism. The human and environment are in mutual process, which is irreversible movement toward greater diversity (Rogers, 1990).

Pattern

Rogers (1992) specifies that the human can be recognized through human field pattern. The human and environment change continuously, yet there is continuity in this ever-changing process. The human pattern and the environmental pattern are rhythmical expressions. These rhythmical expressions are novel, diverse wave patterns. Human energy field pattern is distinguished from the environmental energy field and is perceived as a single wave.

Pandimensionality

Pandimensionality is a "non-linear domain without spatial or temporal attributes" (Rogers, 1992, p. 29). Rogers believes, then, that the unitary human is a pandimensional energy field, recognized by a distinct rhythmical pattern openly changing irreversibly with the pandimensional environmental field.

The principles of helicy, integrality, and resonancy, and the postulates of energy field, openness, pattern, and pandimensionality, along with the existential-phenomenological tenets and concepts, underpin the assumptions about the human and becoming in the human becoming school of thought.

Existential-Phenomenological Tenets and Concepts

Following are the existential-phenomenological tenets of intentionality and human subjectivity and the concepts of coexistence, situated freedom, and coconstitution that are synthesized with Rogers' principles and postulates in the creation of the assumptions of human becoming.

Tenets

The existential-phenomenological tenets of intentionality and human subjectivity evolve from Husserl's belief about the human as unity with the world and Kierkegaard's belief about the human as subject.

Intentionality

This basic tenet posits that the human is by nature an intentional being. This means that the human is open, knows, and is present with the world. To be human, then, is to be intentional and to be involved with the world through a fundamental nature of knowing, being present, and open (Heidegger, 1962, pp. 86-87). The human is involved with the world in creating personal becoming. The creating of personal becoming emerges from the human's historicity and facticity. Human historicity reflects connections with predecessors and contemporaries in creating the who one is at a given moment, and facticity is the immediate situation in which the human finds self. The human is in situation as an already present being and a potential not-yet, open and present with the world. That the human transcends with the present and the possibles bears witness to freedom and the desire to reach beyond. This freedom and desire to reach beyond relate to intentionality in that humans choose in situation a stand with the world and, in so doing, achieve potentials and possibilities all-at-once (Heidegger, 1962, pp. 185-186). This tenet gives rise to the concepts of coexistence and situated freedom.

Human Subjectivity

This basic tenet posits that the human by nature is no thing but, rather, a unity of being with nonbeing—living what is and what is not-yet all-at-once. This means that the human is not a cosmic being or thing in the now but a potential yet-to-be (Heidegger, 1962), a unity of the subject-world changing mutual process. In subjectivity, the human is present with the world in a dialectical relationship (Heidegger, 1962, p. 85), giving meaning to the projects that emerge in the process of becoming. Humans coparticipate with the world in the emergence of projects through choosing to live certain values. This relates to human subjectivity in that the human participates with the world in cocreation of personal becoming. This tenet gives rise to the concept of coconstitution.

Concepts

From the existential-phenomenological tenets of intentionality and human subjectivity emerge these ideas about the human: the human coconstitutes situations with the world, the human experiences existence as coexistence, and the human has freedom in situation.

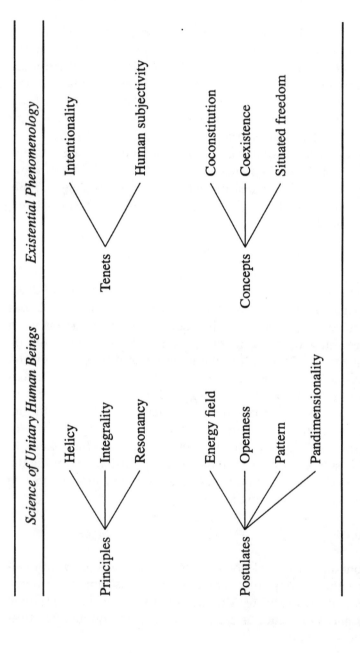

Figure 2.1. Principles, Postulates, Tenets, and Concepts from the Science of Unitary Human Beings and Existential Phenomenology

Coconstitution

The human coconstitutes situations refers to the idea that the meaning emerging in any situation is related to the particular constituents of that situation. The human is enabled and limited by the human-world dialectic through which situations come into being. The human is in mutual process with the various views of the world and others, and indeed cocreates these views by a personal presence (Merleau-Ponty, 1974, pp. 369-409). The human is present with the world and, all-at-once, open to possibilities and, as such, participates in the creation of the world through mutual process (Heidegger, 1962, pp. 252-417).

Coexistence

The human experiences existence as coexistence means that the human is not alone in any dimension of becoming. The human, an emerging being, is with the world with others—predecessors, contemporaries, and successors; indeed, even the act of coming into the world is through others. The human knows becoming in the comprehension of dispersed concrete personal achievements and through the perspectives of others. Without others, one would not know that one is a being. To exist, then, is to coexist as the possibility of transcending to be more than one is, at any given moment (Merleau-Ponty, 1974, pp. 346-365).

Situated Freedom

The human has freedom in situation means that reflectively and prereflectively one participates in choosing the situations in which one finds oneself, as well as one's attitude toward the situations. That is, how a particular situation emerges is related to the human's facticity and to earlier choosings, both those reflected on and those participated in without prior reflection. The human's facticity is that to which the human was born. The givens in situations, then, are present from earlier choosings, from the human's facticity, and the emergent possibilities are cocreated with these givens. The human is a being who can remember past experiences as past events. One creates a personal remembrance by choosing the order and arrangement of reflections on past events as one gives meaning to situations anew. Meanings of the remembered change over time as new experiences shed light on what was as it is appearing now. In choosing ways of being with situations, one incarnates value priorities. The human is compelled to take a stand toward the emergent desires and feelings evolving in situations. One always chooses; as Sartre (1966) says, even "not to choose is in fact to choose not to choose" (p. 619). Choices are made without full knowledge of the outcomes, yet with full responsibility for the consequences.

Figure 2.1 depicts the principles and postulates from the science of unitary human beings and the tenets and concepts from existential-phenomenological thought used in the creation of the assumptions of human becoming.

CHAPTER 3

ASSUMPTIONS ABOUT THE HUMAN AND BECOMING

The principles, tenets, postulates, and concepts from Rogers, Heidegger, Merleau-Ponty, and Sartre described in Chapter 2, "Evolution of the Human Becoming School of Thought," were synthesized in the creation of the assumptions about the human and becoming, underpinning a view of nursing grounded in the human sciences. These assumptions (updated from Parse, 1995, pp. 5-6) follow.

- The human is coexisting while coconstituting rhythmical patterns with the universe.
- The human is open, freely choosing meaning in situation, bearing responsibility for decisions.
- The human is unitary, continuously coconstituting patterns of relating.
- The human is transcending multidimensionally with the possibles.
- Becoming is unitary human-living-health.
- Becoming is a rhythmically coconstituting human-universe process.

- Becoming is the human's patterns of relating value priorities.
- Becoming is an intersubjective process of transcending with the possibles.
- Becoming is unitary human's emerging.

Each assumption is a unique synthesis of the postulates and concepts discussed in Chapter 2: energy field, openness, pattern, pandimensionality, coconstitution, coexistence, and situated freedom.

ASSUMPTION 1:
The Human Is Coexisting While Coconstituting Rhythmical Patterns With the Universe

Assumption 1 is a synthesis of the concepts of coexistence and coconstitution with the postulate pattern. The assumption means that the human lives with others, evolving mutually and in cadence with the universe. The human, a recognizable pattern in the human-universe process, with contemporaries expands the ideas of predecessors positing new notions for successors. This process is the continuity that connects what was with what will be as it is appearing now, bearing witness to human coexistence. To say that the human coexists means that the human lives all-at-once with ancestors, successors, and contemporaries through personal meanings given to others, ideas, objects, situations, and planning projects. That the human coexists with a situation is evidence of participation in coconstituting it. The human coparticipates with the universe in mutually emerging with specific patterns of relating that distinguish the individual from the universe. Patterns of relating are created through the mutual rhythmical human-universe process and incarnate the wholeness of both human and universe. The human, then, is a pattern of patterns of relating distinct from the pattern of the universe. Patterns of relating are the individual's unique ways of being recognized. The human, coexisting with universe, coconstitutes rhythmical patterns of relating.

ASSUMPTION 2:
The Human Is Open, Freely Choosing Meaning in Situation, Bearing Responsibility for Decisions

Assumption 2 is a synthesis of the concept of situated freedom and the postulates of openness and energy field. It means that the human, in open process with the universe, chooses ways of becoming in situation and is accountable for these choices. Unitary human, unique among beings in the universe, appreciates art, music, and moments of joy, and is touched by birthings and dyings, which are the rhythmical happenings of day-to-day living. These happenings are cocreated as the human chooses the meanings of situations and, through these choosings, the possibilities of personal becoming. Choosing meaning incarnates the birthings and dyings inherent in each decision. In choosing one direction, the human gives up others, and in this way is both enabled and limited by the directions chosen and those not chosen. There are enablements and limitations in all decisions. The human incarnates living paradox as being, all-at-once, incarnates nonbeing, that is, living what is and what is not-yet all-at-once. Nonbeing, as a complex phenomenon, can be explained as inherent in being itself. The presence of the human with the universe is the being that surfaces the possibility of nonbeing. The human is aware of the potential of dying or being cut off from the possibility of affirmation in the not-yet. Possibilities for the human arise in the human-universe mutual process. The human and universe, then, in mutual process cocreate situations. The human is responsible for all outcomes of reflective-prereflective choices, even though many are unknown when making decisions.

ASSUMPTION 3:
The Human Is Unitary, Continuously Coconstituting Patterns of Relating

Assumption 3 is a synthesis of the postulates of energy field and pattern and the concept of coconstitution. The human is unitary, different from the sum of parts, and is recognized through ways of becoming, cocreated with the universe. The human as different from the sum of parts means that the human cannot be divided into psychological, biological, sociological, and spiritual components, but, rather, is unitary and recognized as a pattern through individual paradoxical patterns of relating. These are not particulate, but ever-changing, in cocreation with the universe. In mutual process, the pattern of the human emerges with images that incarnate wholeness. These images are unique patterns of relating that are changing and distinguish one human being from another. Coconstituted patterns of relating are unitary human's ways of becoming and are illuminated through speech, words, symbols, silence, gesture, movement, gaze, posture, and touch.

ASSUMPTION 4:
The Human Is Transcending
Multidimensionally With the Possibles

Assumption 4 is a synthesis of the postulates of pandimensionality and openness and the concept of situated freedom. This assumption means that, with the human-universe mutual process, the human chooses to move beyond the actual, the contextual situation, with possibilities. This movement is not repeatable or reversible. The human, in open process, experiences multidimensionally; that is, the human-universe mutual process is lived relatively at many realms of the universe. Space and time are unbounded, nonsequential multidimensional entities. The whole structure of space-time is related to the flow of patterns of interconnections of all that is in the universe. These patterns are the webs of the human-universe process, and are the various universes that the human lives reflectively-prereflectively all-at-once. These webs of interconnections are paradoxal. Paradox implies a unity of apparent opposites; for example, up coexists with down, and hope coexists with no hope. Paradoxical patterns are rhythms with two dimensions; one is usually in the foreground and the other in the background, but they are present all-at-once. In the human-universe process, the human chooses from the many options available in multidimensional experiences. One moves beyond who one is through the mutual human-universe process in imaging possibilities. The imaged possibilities go beyond what is and surface options from which the human chooses a personal becoming. These choices are the new actuals, the contextual situations. The experience of events, then, is related to the relative perspective of the one experiencing them. The new actuals illuminate other possibilities, and the human reaches beyond while continually becoming through choosing. This is the process of transcending with the possibles.

ASSUMPTION 5:
Becoming Is Unitary
Human-Living-Health

Assumption 5 is a synthesis of the postulate of openness and the concepts of situated freedom and coconstitution. This assumption means that, in the human-universe mutual process, there is a continuous movement that both enables and limits becoming. Becoming is the human's continuous changing through mutual process with the universe enhancing diversity. Inherent in changing is choosing who one will be in situation. Choosing is from a unique perspective that is angular and relative, though coconstituted with others. That is, the human's view of the options is from a personal seamless history of becoming. Only the human being living the situation knows it, reflectively and prereflectively. An experience of a situation, although cocreated with others, belongs to one human being only. Choosing some options eliminates others so that possibilities are cocreated and experienced perspectively in the process of becoming—living health. Living health, then, is an incarnation of the human's choosings. It is experienced multidimensionally and lived uniquely, but may be described as relatively sequenced in time, ordered in space, and shared through energy. The unique perspective of each human being's experiencing the human-universe mutual process is health.

ASSUMPTION 6:
Becoming Is a Rhythmically
Coconstituting Human-Universe Process

The concept and postulates synthesized in Assumption 6 are coconstitution, pattern, and pandimensionality. This assumption means that health, the human's becoming, is an undulating process cocreated with human and universe. Becoming is the human's continuous carving out, in cadence with the universe, recognizable patterns of relating. The carving out involves one's changing from what one is to what one wants to be. Changing is an ongoing pulselike rhythm, an ebb and flow of connecting-separating and emerging anew. The connecting-separating phenomenon is a mutual rhythmical paradox. This means that in each connecting, there is also a separating, and with each separating, there is also a connecting. The connections and separations are lived mutually all-at-once. It is this human-universe connecting-separating that coconstitutes the emergence of the human's health as a relative present. The human is always changing multidimensionally, connecting and separating all-at-once. In connecting-separating, the human dwells with particular situations and, through mutual process, new ways of becoming emerge unique to that coming together-moving apart. The human's becoming, then, is the rhythmical process of changing through the mutual connecting-separating of human with universe.

ASSUMPTION 7:
Becoming Is the Human's Patterns
of Relating Value Priorities

Assumption 7 is a synthesis of the concept of situated freedom and the postulates of pattern and openness. This assumption means that becoming is the human's style of living chosen cherished ideals, which are values—prized beliefs. Value priorities are the preferred prized beliefs. Becoming or health is a synthesis of the human's values selected from multidimensional experiences cocreated in mutual process with the universe. The human makes choices from options, affirming as cherished certain ways of becoming. These ways emerge in recognizable patterns and incarnate the human's priorities and changing diversity. These patterns of relating are the human's ways of languaging values and are ever-changing as new values are appropriated. The new values incarnated in day-to-day living emerge as diverse changing priorities. The patterns of relating value priorities constitute the human's becoming.

ASSUMPTION 8:
**Becoming Is an Intersubjective
Process of Transcending With the Possibles**

Assumption 8 is a synthesis of the postulate openness and the concepts situated freedom and coexistence. It means that becoming is moving beyond with the possibles through a subject-to-subject mutual human-universe process. The essence of subject-to-subject experiences originates in coexistence with others, ideas, objects, and situations, and is the human's genuine presence with moment-to-moment emergence. This genuine presence calls forth a risking that is illuminated through the rhythm of revealing-concealing and, thus, reflects the human's choosing diverse ways of becoming. Moving with the possibles means abiding with the familiar while all-at-once struggling with the unfamiliar of an imaged not-yet, as one reveals and conceals who one is and can become. The human's risking is a unitary rhythm of attentively struggling and leaping beyond that propels with diverse possibilities. Becoming is this continuously changing intersubjective process of transcending with the possibles.

ASSUMPTION 9:
Becoming Is Unitary Human's Emerging

The concept and postulates synthesized in this assumption are coexistence, energy field, and pandimensionality. This assumption means that becoming is the human's multidimensional

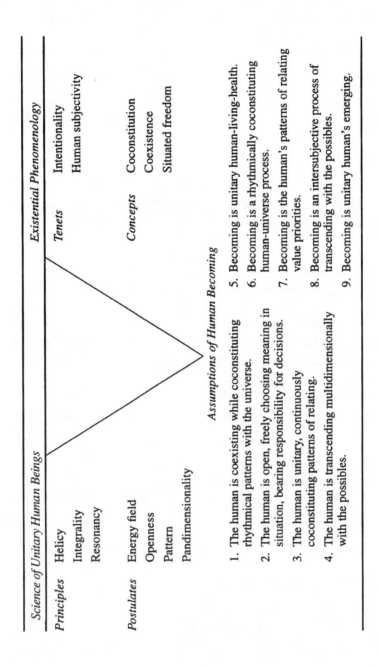

Science of Unitary Human Beings		Existential Phenomenology	
Principles	Helicy	*Tenets*	Intentionality
	Integrality		Human subjectivity
	Resonancy		
Postulates	Energy field	*Concepts*	Coconstitution
	Openness		Coexistence
	Pattern		Situated freedom
	Pandimensionality		

Assumptions of Human Becoming

1. The human is coexisting while coconstituting rhythmical patterns with the universe.
2. The human is open, freely choosing meaning in situation, bearing responsibility for decisions.
3. The human is unitary, continuously coconstituting patterns of relating.
4. The human is transcending multidimensionally with the possibles.
5. Becoming is unitary human-living-health.
6. Becoming is a rhythmically coconstituting human-universe process.
7. Becoming is the human's patterns of relating value priorities.
8. Becoming is an intersubjective process of transcending with the possibles.
9. Becoming is unitary human's emerging.

Figure 3.1. Evolution of Assumptions from Principles, Postulates, Tenets, and Concepts

TABLE 3.1 Interface of Concepts and Postulates With Assumptions

Energy Field Assumptions	Openness Assumptions	Pattern Assumptions	Pandimensionality Assumptions	Coconstitution Assumptions	Coexistence Assumptions	Situated Freedom Assumptions
2	2	1	4	1	1	2
3	4	3	6	3	8	4
9	5	6	9	5	9	5
	7	7		6		7
	8					8

changing in mutual process with the universe. Unitary human's multidimensional experience of coexistence at many realms of the universe powers the creation of individual patterns of relating that arise as rhythms of human becoming. Human health as a nonspecific entity is continuously transforming in diverse ways. Diversity changes with experience, and at any given moment, the human as relative present is different from before and is continuously creating anew, originating uniquely with the ambiguity of the yet-to-be. This means that space-time experiences are not repeatable and are irreversibly integrated with individual patterns of relating. Becoming is the mutual process of human with universe emerging diversely.

Figure 3.1 depicts the relationship of the principles, tenets, postulates, and concepts of Rogers, Heidegger, Sartre, and Merleau-Ponty that were synthesized to form the nine assumptions about the human and becoming.

Each assumption is a synthesis of postulates with concepts in unique three-way combinations. Each of the postulates and concepts explained in Chapter 2, "Evolution of the Human Becoming School of Thought" (energy field, openness, pattern, pandimensionality, coconstitution, coexistence, and situated freedom), is connected at least once with each of the others in the creation of the assumptions of human becoming. Table 3.1 depicts the postulates and concepts with the assumptions in which they appear. Figure 3.2 shows each of the nine assumptions with the relevant postulates and concepts.

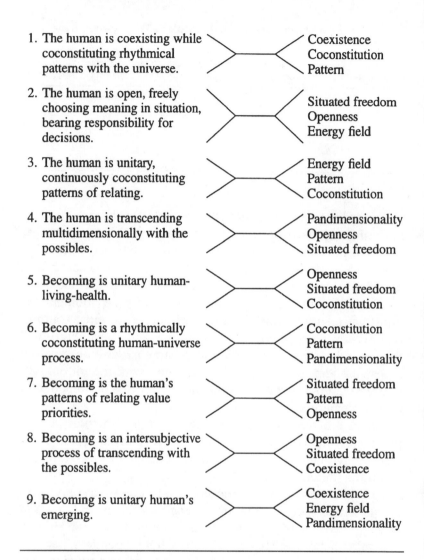

1. The human is coexisting while coconstituting rhythmical patterns with the universe.

   Coexistence
   Coconstitution
   Pattern

2. The human is open, freely choosing meaning in situation, bearing responsibility for decisions.

   Situated freedom
   Openness
   Energy field

3. The human is unitary, continuously coconstituting patterns of relating.

   Energy field
   Pattern
   Coconstitution

4. The human is transcending multidimensionally with the possibles.

   Pandimensionality
   Openness
   Situated freedom

5. Becoming is unitary human-living-health.

   Openness
   Situated freedom
   Coconstitution

6. Becoming is a rhythmically coconstituting human-universe process.

   Coconstitution
   Pattern
   Pandimensionality

7. Becoming is the human's patterns of relating value priorities.

   Situated freedom
   Pattern
   Openness

8. Becoming is an intersubjective process of transcending with the possibles.

   Openness
   Situated freedom
   Coexistence

9. Becoming is unitary human's emerging.

   Coexistence
   Energy field
   Pandimensionality

Figure 3.2. Assumptions With Related Postulates and Concepts

The original nine philosophical assumptions are further synthesized into three assumptions on human becoming (updated from Parse, 1992, p. 38):

- Human becoming is freely choosing personal meaning in situation in the intersubjective process of living value priorities.
- Human becoming is cocreating rhythmical patterns of relating in mutual process with the universe.
- Human becoming is cotranscending multidimensionally with emerging possibles.

The meanings of the philosophical assumptions are not changed through this synthesis. All the assumptions reflect the three major themes: meaning, rhythmicity, and transcendence.

Meaning

There are many denotations and connotations of the term *meaning*. Definitions include *essence, trend, intention, significance,* and many others. Dilthey (1961) believes that meaning is what expressions express and understanding understands. He says that to have meaning, an expression must point beyond itself. Meanings are the valued images of the is, was, and will-be languaged in the now with and without words, with and without movement. Meaning refers to the linguistic and imagined content of something and the interpretation that one gives to something. It arises with the human-universe process and refers to ultimate meaning or purpose in life and the meaning moments of everyday living. Meaning moments change through the living of new experiences that shift imaged values, shedding a different light and thus changing ultimate meaning. Meaning, then, is not static but ever-changing, and thus portends the unknown, the yet-to-be truths for the moment. "Meaning is both personal and shared, both representation and event, and all these without boundaries" (Cody, 1994, p. 50).

Rhythmicity

Rhythmicity is the cadent, paradoxical patterning of the human-universe mutual process. Unrepeatable rhythmical patterns are revealed and concealed all-at-once with a flowing process as cadences change with new experiences arising with diversity. The patterns are paradoxical in that they are not opposites but, rather, dimensions of the same rhythm lived all-at-once. They are ever-shifting with the emergence of the differences in change and the continuity of persistence all-at-once. The rhythmical patterns are recognizable configurations of human with universe. Human with universe connects and separates all-at-once with others, ideas, objects, and situations, and is enabled and limited by the infinite numbers of opportunities and restrictions inherent in all choosings.

Transcendence

Transcendence is reaching beyond with possibles—the hopes and dreams envisioned in multidimensional experiences. The possibles arise with the human-universe process as options from which to choose personal ways of becoming. Transcendence is powering the originating of transforming. The human propels with the creation of new ventures, as struggling and leaping beyond shift the views of the now, expanding horizons and bringing to light other possibles.

These three themes—meaning, rhythmicity, and transcendence—each lead to one of the principles. Meaning is the central theme of the principle on structuring meaning multidimensionally. Rhythmicity is the central theme of the principle on cocreating rhythmical patterns, and transcendence is the central theme of cotranscending with the possibles.

CHAPTER 4

PRINCIPLES, CONCEPTS, AND THEORETICAL STRUCTURES OF HUMAN BECOMING

The assumptions about the human and becoming posited as the foundation of this theory of nursing rooted in the human sciences are explained in Chapter 3, "Assumptions About the Human and Becoming." The human is postulated as unitary, mutually cocreating with the universe rhythmical paradoxical patterns of relating. The unitary human freely chooses meaning in situation, bears responsibility for the choices, and transcends with possibles.

Human becoming as a theory emerges from the assumptions. Human becoming is a unitary phenomenon that refers to the human's cocreation of rhythmical patterns of relating in mutual process with the universe. The words *human becoming* form a construct reflecting a conceptual bond that points to human quality of life and health as ongoing mutual participation with the universe. *Quality of life* is the incarnation of lived experiences in the indivisible human's views on living moment to moment (becoming) as the changing patterns of shifting perspectives weave the fabric of life through the human-universe process

(Parse, 1994c). Only this definition of quality of life is consistent with the human becoming school of thought, but many authors have defined it from different perspectives (see Parse, 1994c). The human's *health* is becoming; it is not a linear entity that can be interrupted or qualified by terms such as *good, bad, more,* or *less.* It is not adapting to or coping with the environment; such a description of health dichotomizes and denies the human's unitary nature and mutual process with the universe. Unitary human's health is a synthesis of values, a way of living.

Health is defined by many authors, and some definitions are consistent with the ontology of human becoming. Goldstein (1959) describes health as a value chosen by the human. He believes that this value is a characteristic of true being; in fact, it is reflective of the human-universe mutual process. Dubos (1979b) supports the idea that values and attitudes are related to the human's health, and that health itself transcends cause-effect relationships. Consistent with this idea is Frankl's (1967) belief that health as a value emerges as the human continually structures meaning in situation. This points to human becoming as a process. Dubos (1979a) says health is "not a state but a potentiality" (p. 395). This is congruent with van Kaam's (1974) view of the whole of human development. He says,

> As man I am both "potentiality" and "emergence" . . . I experience my potentiality as a dynamic tendency toward self emergence. I am not only what I actually am; I am also a constant movement towards self emergence. . . . I am "becoming." I am the potentiality of dying to my life at any moment and to being born to what I am not yet. (pp. 109-110)

Consistent with this view is Ferguson's (1980) suggestion of an emergent paradigm of health, the assumptions of which include health as a view of the whole person with an emphasis on human values and caring. Dossey (1982) suggests a space-time model of health that specifies health as human connectedness, and LeShan (1982) believes health is a whole-person phenomenon and healing is a process of the person's total life. Serge King (1981) says that individuals have only the limitations they agree to have and that health is a choice. Mann (1997) states that "we are living at a time of paradigm shift in thinking about health. . . . Health as well-being, despite the World Health Organization's definition, lacks more than rudimentary definition" (p. 13). Other authors from various disciplines and in different works have continued to foster this view of health consistent with the human becoming perspective, in which human health is considered a reflection of individual choice and value priorities (Chopra, 1989, 1993; Cousins, 1983, 1989; Dacher, 1997; Dossey, 1982, 1984, 1991, 1993; Liberman, 1991; Moyers, 1993; Siegel, 1989; Sontag, 1979; Weil, 1995).

Health from the human becoming perspective is not the opposite of disease or a state that the human has but, rather, a continuously changing process that the human cocreates in mutual process with the universe. This notion was substantiated in the findings from a phenomenological study on health (Parse, Coyne, & Smith, 1985), with 400 participants between the ages of 7 and 93 who were asked to describe their experiences of health. Descriptions by the participants showed that the experience of health is much more than the absence of disease and more than a dynamic state of well-being; it is a harmony sparked by energy arising with plenitude, cocreated by the person in mutual process with the universe. Health is a personal commitment that each person lives incarnating his or her own value priorities (Parse, 1990a). The personal commitment is lived through abiding with the struggles and joys of everydayness. The way of abiding with the joys and struggles of everydayness is the choosing of meaning in situations at the reflective-prereflective realms of the universe. This is health. Disease from the human becoming perspective is not something a person contracts but, rather, a pattern of the human-universe mutual process.

All patterns of human becoming are recognized through languaging the cocreated paradoxical processes (revealing-concealing, enabling-limiting, and connecting-separating) that emerge in transcending with imagined valued possibles. In structuring meaning, the human freely chooses in situation ways of originating while emerging with the possibles. Emerging with the possibles is powering ways of transforming with diversity, incarnating chosen values from options envisioned in multidimensional experiences. Human becoming, then, is structuring meaning multidimensionally in cocreating paradoxical rhythmical patterns of relating while cotranscending with the possibles. The specific principles of human becoming are structuring meaning multidimensionally, cocreating rhythmical patterns of relating, and cotranscending with the possibles. The three concepts in each principle are stated in verbal forms to express more clearly the idea of human becoming as an ongoing changing process.

- Structuring meaning multidimensionally is cocreating reality through the languaging of valuing and imaging.
- Cocreating rhythmical patterns of relating is living the paradoxical unity of revealing-concealing and enabling-limiting while connecting-separating.
- Cotranscending with the possibles is powering unique ways of originating in the process of transforming.

These principles bring to light the idea of living paradox (Mitchell, 1993; Parse, 1981, 1994c) as fundamental to human becoming. A paradox is an apparent opposite. In the human becoming theory, a paradox is considered to be one phenomenon with two dimensions. Paradoxes are not problems to be solved or eliminated, but are natural rhythms of life. Living paradox is "a rhythmical shifting of views, the awareness of which arises through experiencing the contradiction of opposites in the day-to-day relating of value priorities while journeying to the not-yet" (Mitchell, 1993, p. 44).

Principle 1 has the paradox of explicit-tacit knowing of imaging. Explicit knowing is that which is known reflectively and is utterable. Tacit knowing is prereflective unutterable knowing. Explicit-tacit knowing is lived reflectively-prereflectively all-at-once (Parse, 1981, 1994c). The confirming-not confirming of valuing is the persistent living of what is cherished and not cherished all-at-once. Speaking-being silent and moving-being still are paradoxical rhythms of languaging (Parse, 1994c). Principle 2 clearly specifies the paradoxes in the concepts revealing-concealing, enabling-limiting, and connecting-separating. Principle 3 also has paradoxical rhythms connected with each concept. The pushing-resisting of powering is the mutually forging and holding that enlivens the ebb and flow of life, and being-nonbeing is all-at-once living the now and the unknown not-yet. The affirming-not-affirming paradox is all-at-once living reverence amid disregard. The conformity-nonconformity of originating is the all-at-once movement to be like others and yet unique. The paradox certainty-uncertainty is all-at-once being sure and unsure in choosing among options. The familiar-unfamiliar of transforming refers to the all-at-once transfiguring of an unfamiliar perspective to the familiar, as others, ideas, objects, and situations are viewed in a new light.

PRINCIPLE 1:
Structuring Meaning Multidimensionally Is Cocreating Reality Through the Languaging of Valuing and Imaging

This principle means that human becoming is the ongoing constructing of reality through assigning significance to experiences at the many realms of the universe that are lived all-at-once. For each person, an infinite number of realms exists in mutual process, in that reality is a seamless symphony of becoming, the timeless moments of one's history, the was, is, and will-be all-at-once (Parse, 1996a). The timeless moments are nontemporal and refer to the all-at-once incarnation of meaning (Ricoeur, 1984, 1985, 1988). Meaning surfaces as reality is made concrete through a person's choices (Toben, 1975). In the human-universe process, one chooses from the many options, emerging with multidimensional experiences as one constructs a personal reality. This personal reality incarnates all that a person is, has been, and will become all-at-once (Dilthey, 1961). Humans are not given reality but have to construct it for themselves in their own way (Whorf, 1956), "for there is nothing either good or bad, but thinking makes it so" (Shakespeare, 1600/1978). Constructing reality is giving meaning to unique experiences (Toben, 1975). Meaning refers to the meaning moments of every day and the ultimate meaning of purposes in life. Each unique experience stretches meaning moments beyond what is and sheds new light expanding ultimate meaning. Unique experiences are the individual's perspectives incarnated through the personal languaging of imaging and valuing. Imaging, valuing, and languaging are the concepts of structuring meaning multidimensionally.

Imaging

Imaging, the first concept of structuring meaning multidimensionally, is reflective-prereflective coming to know the explicit-tacit all-at-once. Reality is constructed through this mutual reflective-prereflective process that is the shaping of personal knowledge explicitly-tacitly. In the explicit-tacit paradox, explicit knowing is articulated logically and reflected on critically. It has form and substance, and tacit knowing is prereflective—prearticulate and acritical—"the unreasoned conclusions of our senses" (Polanyi, 1959, p. 17). Tacit knowing is quiet and vague and lies hidden from reflective awareness, somewhat anonymous. The human is a questioning being, however, and all that is imaged explicitly-tacitly is an answer to a question, and the questioning is a searching for certainty in knowing.

> Knowing—that is, picturing [imaging] "the world" to ourselves is not a purely intellectual affair. . . . Our active attitude makes a difference. . . . There are no pure events for us—no "facts" uncontaminated by the influence of our knowing activities; there are only events colored by and situated in the context of our previously accepted ideas-feelings-beliefs-behavior. (Bruteau, 1979, p. 35)

Explicit-tacit knowing emerges mutually through abiding with, comparing, and appropriating the subsidiary awareness of particulars with the focal awareness of wholes, thus cocreating the indivisible meanings of experiences (Polanyi, 1969, p. 134). Appropriating new ideas with a worldview is through "utilization of a framework for unfolding our understanding in accordance with the indications and standards imposed by the framework" (Polanyi, 1969, p. 134).

For example, one confronted for the first time with the notion that the human is different from the sum of parts examines the idea in light of personal knowledge about the human, which is that the human is the sum of parts. One compares the new idea with the standards of one's personal framework to see whether or not the idea is compatible. If the idea is compatible, the person may incarnate it with the repertoire of knowledge, expanding horizons of personal knowing. If it is not, the person may disregard the notion or, if convinced that the idea is worthy, may alter the standards of the framework to include this idea. The process of reflective-preflective abiding with others, ideas, objects, and situations, comparing the new with personal beliefs, and appropriating, then, is how humans structure meaning through cocreating personal reality. Schutz (1967) writes, "The meaning of our experiences . . . constitutes reality" (pp. 209-212). Greene (1978) says that "to talk of meaning is to talk of interpretation. . . . It is to allow for the fact that there are multiple realities available to human consciousness and a network of relationships to effect that have much to do with the living self" (p. 16). She further says that "the province of science, art, play or dream—is composed of a sect [sic] of more or less compatible experiences. . . . [and always] . . . interpreted in accord with a characteristic cognitive style" (p. 16).

The significance one gives to an event, then, is a reflection of the whole person (Dilthey, 1961; Harman, 1997; Heidegger, 1962). This means that one structures reflectively-prereflectively meanings compatible with one's worldview—the history of one's choosings in the was and will-be as they are appearing now. Imaging reality, making concrete the meaning of multidimensional experiences, then, incarnates the mutuality of the explicit-implicit knowing and is an essential feature of human becoming.

Valuing

Valuing, the second concept of structuring meaning multidimensionally, is confirming-not confirming cherished beliefs in light of a personal worldview. The paradoxical rhythm of confirming-not confirming is choosing from imaged options and owning the choices. The cherished choosings are integrated with one's value framework, which is a matrix of principles and ideas that guide one's life. The matrix screens all that is imaged with one's multidimensional experiences.

According to Raths, Harmin, and Simon (1978), there are seven essentials in the valuing process. An attitude or belief becomes a value for a person when these seven essentials are present: choosing freely, choosing from alternatives, reflectively choosing, prizing and cherishing, affirming, acting on choices, and repeating. The three key activities in the valuing process, then, are choosing, prizing, and acting. B. P. Hall (1976) concurs with Raths et al. when he says,

> To value is to make a choice and act upon it. The choices and acts of one constitute one's history. But as one chooses and acts on values, one also seeks meaning—meaning making and valuing are for all intents and purposes aspects of the same reality. (p. 3)

Hall further states that "the act of valuing is the stance the self takes toward the environment such that the self acquires meaning, and the creative development of both the self and the environment is enhanced" (p. 26).

Creating reality, then, is giving meaning to imaged multidimensional experiences through valuing. A value is a symbol that signifies meaning. For example, a couple adopts a child. This action reflects a prizing of sharing their lives with children. This value was chosen from options available in their multidimensional experiences. The living of this value structures the meaning of family for the couple. Another example is a person who changes food-intake patterns to reduce weight to present a lean, attractive appearance. This action reflects a prizing, obviously, for presenting a lean, attractive appearance, and is a value chosen from options in the person's multidimensional experiences. In these examples, the couple valued having children more than living alone together, and the person valued an attractive, lean look more than eating to excess. Both of these values reflect choosing, prizing, and acting to beliefs. Appropriating a new value is struggling with a decision to confirm a cherished belief while not confirming others; it is choosing one while all-at-once giving up others.

Through the valuing process, new beliefs are continuously being examined; some are appropriated and integrated with those values held as cherished and others are not. The ever-changing values reflect a person's expanding diversity. A synthesis of values is one's health. Through choosing valued images from multidimensional experiences, humans structure meaning as a feature of human becoming.

Languaging

Languaging, the third concept of structuring meaning multidimensionally, is signifying valued images through speaking-being silent and moving-being still. This means that the cocreated images one chooses as values give unique meaning to multidimensional experiences and are symbolized through languaging. One's way of languaging emerges with the human-universe process as one's structuring of reality (Bandler & Grinder, 1975a, 1975b; Ricoeur, 1987; Watzlawick, 1978). It is reflective of the interconnectedness of humans from generation to generation (Gadamer, 1993; E. T. Hall, 1976). People in close association who have common ties and interests cocreate and perpetuate language and living patterns; thus, although unique realities are structured by each individual, these are cocreated through mutual process with others. It is through languaging that each individual symbolizes unique realities, since language is always personal (Whorf, 1956). This symbolizing surfaces in speaking-being silent and moving-being still. Speaking-being silent is a paradoxical process of "vocal actualization of the tendency to see realities symbolically" (Sapir, 1966, p. 15), and quiet contemplation in the deep place of no words that symbolizes much (Parse, 1997a). Moving-being still, another paradoxical process of languaging, is a symbolic mode of signifying meaning. "Moving, like speaking, is a sign or symbol expressing meaning" (Sapir, 1966, p. 72). Being still is a near motionless stance that appears to be like treading water in one place, yet it is not. It is a clear expression of the meaning of the moment. The meaning signified is one's patterns of relating the symbols of words and no words through tonality, tempo, and volume, as well as gesture, gaze, touch, and posture (Gadamer, 1993; von Bertalanffy, 1959).

These symbols are lived all-at-once in the human-universe process. When one person greets another person, rhythmical patterns of relating emerge as words become sentences and are shared with a certain volume at a particular tempo with unique intonation, all-at-once with a certain gaze, gesture, touch, and posture. Languaging is not just the content of what a person says with words, but how the whole message is uncovered in the context of the situation. It is the rhythmical moments of silence, the choice of words and syntax, the intonation, the facial expressions, the gestures, the posture, and that which is not said and movements that are not made that constitute the symbolic expression characteristic of languaging as a concept of structuring meaning multidimensionally. Languaging is "the intention to unveil the thing itself and go beyond what is said [through speaking-being silent and moving-being still] to what what is said signifies" (Merleau-Ponty, 1973, p. 102). The signification, that is, the meaning, is made concrete in the content and structure of the sentences (Gadamer, 1993; Ricoeur, 1985, 1987, 1988, 1992; Straus, 1974) and in the gestures, intonations, facial expressions, and silences (Parse, 1981, 1992).

Themes emerge in being with others, and personal projects make clear individuals' valued images. The meanings that surface all-at-once in a given situation emerge from the context of the situation with the intent and history of the individuals coconstituting the moment (Dossey, 1991; Parse, 1981, 1992, 1995). Each individual is languaging unique imaged values and is sharing with others a worldview that is the incarnation of a personal history and specific intention in cocreating the context of the event. Worldview is world image. "World image is the most comprehensive, most complex synthesis of myriads of experiences . . . the . . . ascription of value and meaning . . . a pattern of patterns" (Watzlawick, 1978, p. 43). In the rhythm of human-human presence, individuals give messages consistent with personal valued images. The message the other receives is all-at-once, yet not complete. Full understanding of the message is not possible in light of the realms of knowing, that is, the explicit-tacit knowing, what is known and utterable and what is known and not utterable (Gadamer, 1993; Parse, 1981, 1995). No individual can fully understand another; each experiences the other from a personal perspective (E. T. Hall, 1976, p. 69). As Grinder and Bandler (1976) say, "the map is not the territory" (p. 4).

The individual is the whole territory, full of the ambiguity and mystery always present in human involvements. The map is only the blueprint, without the intricacies of the human process. The sharing of worldviews through speaking-being silent and moving-being still is a complex process in that each individual experiences from a unique perspective, and this perspective is never the same as it is for the others. Interpretations are meanings arising from experiencing the other and are always perspectival (Gadamer, 1993; Parse, 1981; Ricoeur, 1985, 1987, 1988, 1992).

Perspective or worldview is not embedded in the context of the situation but, rather, emerges mutually with the languaging of chosen imaged values in the human-universe process. "What [the human] chooses is what gives structure and meaning to his [or her] world" (E. T. Hall, 1976, p. 88). For example, individuals experiencing a given event describe the details of the event differently, though there may be common themes in the description. The differences arise with the unique imaging of values as languaged by each person. Languaging imaged values is creating reality in the process of structuring meaning and is a recognizable feature of human becoming.

Weaving a "fabric of meaning" (Langer, 1976, p. 266) as one's life, then, is structuring meaning multidimensionally through imaging, valuing, and languaging. Meaning is continuously changing as the individual changes, incarnating diverse patterns, as different images give rise to possibilities for appropriating new values with original languaging. Structuring meaning multidimensionally is seen in everyday life experiences as an identifiable manifestation of human becoming.

For example, Bill and Mary decided to get married, creating the Abrams family. Both Bill and Mary had imaged many possibilities for themselves before making the decision. One example is their choosing to integrate their family backgrounds to form a new reality for themselves. Mary's family heritage was quite different from Bill's. She had few opportunities to continue her education, and making money was highly valued by her parents. Bill's family, on the other hand, of different ethnic background, placed great significance on status and education. Bill's family was unhappy with his choice of Mary as a bride. Both Bill and Mary shared their family's values somewhat; but, in sharing each other's worldviews on many issues, they imaged other ways of being together and chose the valuing of each other in a marital relationship. Each, through dwelling with and appropriating some of the other's worldviews, cocreated the reality of Mr. and Mrs. Abrams. They chose from alternatives, prized each other, and acted on the chosen alternative. They languaged through symbols such as a wedding announcement, wedding rings, and living together, making concrete their imaged values for each other. The structuring of meaning multidimensionally is exemplified in the decision of Bill and Mary to create the Abrams family, and this is the incarnation of their becoming.

PRINCIPLE 2:
Cocreating Rhythmical Patterns of Relating
Is Living the Paradoxical Unity of Revealing-Concealing
and Enabling-Limiting While Connecting-Separating

This principle means that human becoming is an emerging cadence of coconstituting ways of becoming with the universe. These ways of becoming (revealing-concealing, enabling-limiting, and connecting-separating) are paradoxical, lived rhythmically, and recognized in the human-universe process as patterns. They are paradoxical in that they appear to be opposites, but are really two dimensions of the same rhythm present all-at-once. One dimension is in the foreground, the other is in the background. Their rhythmicity is reflected in the diversity of patterns arising with change.

To say that the human's patterns of relating are rhythmical means that they have qualities of timing and flowing (Leonard, 1978). Timing refers to the cadence evident in a recurrent beat. It is sometimes fast, sometimes slow, but ever-emerging universally. Flowing refers to the continuity evident as the changing beats incarnate diverse patterns, like waves of the sea, moving with the alternating rise and fall, somewhat the same yet becoming different with each movement of wave with wave and wave with sea. Timing and flowing are evident in the rhythmical patterns of human becoming. For example, as person-to-person engagements become more frequent between two or more individuals, the rhythm changes with each meeting, cocreating diverse patterns in that each individual has emerged through other experiences since their last meeting. Rhythmical patterns of relating are paradoxical and are lived all-at-once in situation.

For example, a person may choose to live joy in the foreground with a dying loved one, while the inevitable sorrow is all-at-once present in the background. In this situation, the person with the dying loved one reveals-conceals, is enabled-limited, and connects-separates all-at-once. The specific concepts of this principle are paradoxical rhythms of human becoming: revealing-concealing, enabling-limiting, and connecting-separating.

Revealing-Concealing

Revealing-concealing is disclosing-not disclosing all-at-once. Fundamental to this rhythm is the notion of the human as mystery—an appreciation of the unexplainable in human becoming. For Buber (1965), the idea of disclosing-not disclosing is related to being and seeming, the duality of the interhuman. Being is the way a human knows self; seeming is the way the human portrays self to others (Buber, 1965). Buber believes the human chooses to reveal and conceal all-at-once in mutual process with others. There is always more to a person than what the other experiences in the immediate situation; there is always that which is all-at-once concealed.

Marcel (1978) agrees with Buber when he discusses presence. He says there is always mystery present, that which cannot be readily ascertained about a person, that which is hidden. Jourard (1971) concurs with Buber and Marcel when he discusses disclosing and not-disclosing as the way the human relates to others. He believes that self-disclosure involves courage, and in the process of becoming known to another, one gains knowledge of self (Jourard, 1971). The rhythm of disclosing-not disclosing for Jourard is involved with choosing and being authentic and is a reflection of health. For Gadamer (1993), what one discloses or does not disclose in conversation cannot be determined prior to engagement: "No one knows in advance what will 'come out' of a conversation" (p. 383). This reflects the view that all process is cocreated with the constituents of a situation. The rhythmical pattern of revealing-concealing flows in cadence, human with universe, as a recognizable feature of human becoming.

Enabling-Limiting

Enabling-limiting is living the opportunities-restrictions present in all choosings all-at-once. In choosing, the human moves in one direction, which restricts movement in another, and there are both opportunities and restrictions in what is chosen and opportunities and restrictions in what is not chosen. Sartre (1966) believes that the human is fundamentally free and chooses to be certain ways in situation. These ways are always enabling-limiting. The human continuously makes choices; every event in the universe is an opportunity to choose. Merleau-Ponty (1974) agrees with Sartre, and he states that the human is "open to an infinite number of possibilities" (p. 453). But the human cannot be all possibilities at once, so, in choosing, one is both enabled and limited. A recognizable flow and cadence emerge with the enabling-limiting of human becoming.

Connecting-Separating

Connecting-separating is being with and apart from others, ideas, objects, and situations all-at-once. It is discussed by a number of theorists, who generally give this rhythmical pattern similar meaning but name it differently. Unifying and separating is a happening, according to Kempler (1974), who believes that each separating leads to a higher order of union, and the process of separating and unifying is the "main thrust of human development" (p. 65).

Buber (1965) concurs with Kempler (1974) in a general sense. Buber's view is that a twofold principle of human life is distancing and relating. He believes that one can enter into a relationship only with that which one has set at a distance. When relating with one phenomenon, others are set at a distance. van Kaam, van Croonenburg, and Muto (1969) say that the human "is a rhythm of communion and aloneness" (p. 30). Both aspects of connecting-separating are a source of human emergence. Communion is being involved with the activity at hand while all-at-once not being involved, and being involved in a way with other activities. Moving away from the activity at hand is all-at-once moving with and away from other activities. For example, when two or more people come together in an intersubjective process, that is, they are truly present to each other, they all-at-once are separating from others, yet in their connecting there is an all-at-once separating, and in the separation there is a connection. This rhythmic pattern confirms the human as uniquely connecting-separating all-at-once. In everyday living, the human is all-at-once close to some phenomena and distant from others. In closeness, there is also distance, and in distance, there is a closeness. This is a continuous cadent process and a feature of human becoming.

The rhythmical patterns of relating—revealing-concealing, enabling-limiting, and connecting-separating—are seen in everyday life experiences as identifiable manifestations of human becoming. For example, Mr. and Mrs. Baker and their children, 15-year-old Jim and 10-year-old Sharon, have chosen to jog together twice a week. This activity is a way of connecting the family as a unit while separating the family from other persons and phenomena. Within the family method of jogging, such as who runs next to whom, there can also be seen a connection of two or more family members while all-at-once a separation from others. The family running session enables and limits all-at-once in that it enables family togetherness while limiting other activities for its members, perhaps golf, swimming, or football. The choosing of one activity for now limits participating in another. Jogging together as a family reveals a value for jogging and being together, but all-at-once conceals the value for other activities as well as the meaning of jogging and being together for each family member. Cocreating rhythmical patterns of relating is exemplified in the Baker family's jogging together, and this is an incarnation of human becoming.

PRINCIPLE 3:
Cotranscending With the Possibles Is Powering Unique Ways of Originating in the Process of Transforming

This principle means that human becoming is moving beyond with intended hopes and dreams while pushing-resisting in creating new ways of viewing the familiar and unfamiliar (Parse, 1992). The human aspires and reaches beyond to that which is not-yet (Merleau-Ponty, 1974). This reaching beyond does not mean beyond experience; it means living with the various realms of experience all-at-once (Marcel, 1978). The human exists with others and continues to cocreate new possibles that arise from the context of situations as opportunities from which alternatives are chosen. The contexts of situations are present from prior choosings and cocreate other possibles, and, in this way, the human continuously invents ways of becoming while cotranscending with the possibles.

Human existence is such that the human is coconstituting the situation and all-at-once cotranscending with it. Through multidimensional experiences, the human is aware of other possibles from which free choices in situation can be made.

> By transcending the given situation . . . [the human] frees himself
> within certain limits from the situation. This opens up alternatives;
> the dimension of actuality is left behind and the realm of potenti-
> ality is entered, creating the possibility of choice and the necessity
> of decision. (Weisskopf, 1959, p. 109)

The human's orientation with the possible is in powering and cocreating that which is beyond the moment in indefinite space-time (Merleau-Ponty, 1963).

Cotranscending with the possibles, then, is the way the human with the universe reaches and propels beyond (Frankl, 1959), cocreating anew in the changing of change. The concepts of cotranscending with the possibles are powering, originating, and transforming.

Powering

Powering is the pushing-resisting process of affirming-not affirming being in light of nonbeing. "It originates when we turn toward the future which happens in different ways; in dreams of future happiness, in the play of imagination with possibilities, in hesitations, and in fear" (Dilthey, 1961, p. 109). Since human orientation is toward the future, powering is fundamental to being (Tillich, 1954). It is the force of human existence and underpins the courage to be (Tillich, 1952). That the human exists means that the human is powering. One cannot not power. Powering is a human-universe process recognized in a continuous affirming-not affirming of being in the presence of the possibility of nonbeing. Being is in paradoxical apposition with nonbeing. Nonbeing arises in everyday life as humans all-at-once live what is with the unknown not-yet. The nonbeing is the not-yet known and the potential risk of losing something of value. The risk refers not only to dying but to being rejected, threatened, or not recognized in a manner consistent with expectations. The risks arise in the birthings and dyings of everyday moments lived with the ambiguity of what is about to be. Powering is a continuous rhythmical process incarnating intentions and actions in moving with possibilities. Pushing-resisting is an essential rhythm of powering all-at-once "in every moment of life in all relations of all beings . . . between [human] and nature, between [human] and [human], between individuals and groups, between groups and groups" (Tillich, 1954, p. 42).

Pushing-resisting patterns emerge in the human-universe process and are present in every human engagement, creating tension and sometimes conflict. Possibles emerge through the tension and conflict that create alternatives from which one can choose in reaching beyond. Tension is the struggling between pushing and resisting while engaging with others, issues, ideas, desires, and hopes all-at-once in striving to reach new possibles. In the struggling, an individual cotranscends with what is not-yet.

Conflict surfaces in situation when the tension between pushing and resisting is changed, opening the way for opposition between and among worldviews relative to issues. Conflict offers opportunities for individuals to examine the worldviews of others in situation and to make choices with others to move beyond with new possibles. Powering is a process in all change, as one moves from what one is to what one is not-yet.

For example, the Cook family, a husband and wife with one child, have a pattern of relating in which Mrs. Cook makes decisions and Mr. Cook generally agrees. They discover, after living the tension of pushing-resisting, that their worldviews differ about their child's discipline relative to scholastic performance. Mrs. Cook believes strongly in using incentives such as extra money and new material acquisitions to encourage better scholastic performance; this becomes the course of action with the child and Mr. Cook quietly agrees. The Cook family lives the pushing-resisting tension pattern for a period of time. Mrs. Cook continually encourages the child to perform better through offering material goods. This is pushing, emphasizing her worldview, while at the same time it is a resisting of her husband's view. Mr. Cook's silence is pushing, in that it pushes Mrs. Cook to continue the discipline strategy. He is all-at-once resisting the opportunity to initiate a new struggle and change the discipline strategy. These individual powering patterns of Mr. and Mrs. Cook with their child emerge in the day-to-day living of this decision. Mr. Cook, who quietly agreed to the arrangement, remains silent while Mrs. Cook struggles in conversation with the child relative to the rewards for scholastic performance. Mrs. Cook, whose idea it was to discipline in this way, experiences frustration. Mr. Cook remains silent, and the struggle of powering with powering is apparent until the child's scholastic performance becomes an issue for the parents. Mr. Cook decides to participate no longer in the original decision of remaining silent. The pushing-resisting rhythm is changed, and conflict surfaces. The parents confront their worldviews as different and new alternatives arise, such as restricting the child, combining restricting and incentives, as well as others. The new possibles bring to the surface new ways of viewing the situation, and powering struggles with powering as each parent affirms and all-at-once does not affirm being with nonbeing, that is, living with the unknown of what is not-yet and the threat of not having his or her own values lived in the family. Through this struggle, the family cotranscends with what is not-yet. In this way, powering is an essence of cotranscending with the possibles. It is an everyday occurrence and a recognizable feature of human becoming.

Originating

Originating is inventing new ways of conforming-not conforming in the certainty-uncertainty of living. It is creating ways of distinguishing personal uniqueness (Nietzsche, 1968) by living the paradoxical rhythms of conformity-nonconformity and certainty-uncertainty all-at-once. Conformity-nonconformity surfaces in the human-universe process, as individuals seek to be like others, yet, all-at-once, not to be like others. Seeking to be like others is to focus on commonalties, while seeking to be different is to focus on that which is uniquely distinct. The paradox of living certainty-uncertainty surfaces in the human-universe process as individuals make clear their choices in situation yet, all-at-once, live the ambiguity of the unknown outcomes; the sure-unsure exists all-at-once. Individuals are called on continuously by others to be more conforming and less unique, while moving with that which is more certain than uncertain; when each defines conformity and certainty in the same way, then all strive for commonness. There may be more comfort in sameness and more safety in certainty.

The kind of certainty-uncertainty and conformity-nonconformity, not the degree, is significant in patterns of originating. One does not have more or less certainty or conformity but, rather, certainty and conformity arise in the context of the situation as ways of becoming in situation are chosen. Originating, then, springs from cotranscending with these paradoxes in day-to-day living. To transcend with the paradoxes, one imagines new possibles, thus opening up "vast opportunities for inventing novel connections and seeing unusual analogies" (Bruteau, 1979, p. 219) for originating transformation. With a particular decision, one seeks a vision of the whole structure, a completed picture of what living the decision would mean, that is, creative imagining (Parse, 1990a). The vision of the whole structure moves one to be more comfortable with the unique, thus living the paradoxical unity of conformity-nonconformity. The idea of the whole structure also moves one to make clear choices while anticipating the outcomes, yet with the ambiguity of not knowing the actual outcomes in living the paradox of certainty-uncertainty. The process of originating is coconstituted with the human-universe process. Conformity-nonconformity and certainty-uncertainty are patterns of originating in situation.

For example, Mr. and Mrs. Daly and their son, Mike, are confronted with the decision of choosing a university for Mike. In the decision making relative to this issue, the family patterns of originating surface. The family has many options, because Mike is an acceptable candidate for many universities. From the many options, the family cocreates the image, the whole structure of Mike attending an Ivy League school. This moves the Daly family to be comfortable in seeking some common ground with Ivy League families, while being comfortable as a unique and autonomous family, living conformity-nonconformity all-at-once. Mike would be the only member of his graduating class and his generational family to attend an Ivy League school. The whole structure with the visioned outcomes—Mike would perform well enough to remain in school; investments would be lucrative enough to finance his education; and the family's social class would be enhanced—moves the family to apply for Mike's admission, knowing the ambiguity relative to the various possible outcomes. This is living the paradox of certainty-uncertainty. Through this process of originating, the family changes as it invents new ways of living the patterns of conformity-nonconformity and certainty-uncertainty. In this way, originating is an essence of cotranscending with the possibles and is a recognizable feature of human becoming.

Transforming

Transforming is shifting the view of the familiar-unfamiliar, the changing of change in coconstituting anew in a deliberate way. In the human-universe process, change is ongoing; that is, the human coparticipates with the universe in mutual emergence. This emergence arises as the human with the universe cocreates becoming. Deliberate innovative discoveries and shifts in worldview are also coconstituted through mutual process as the human attends to discoveries, and the phenomena are available to be discovered. This idea is supported by van den Berg (1971) in his theory of changes. van den Berg believes that discoveries surfacing at a given moment are directly related to both the ongoing changes in human existence and the all-at-once changes in the world over time. He believes in a person-world "changeable togetherness" (p. 288) that in itself surfaces unique possibilities for discovery.

Unique possibilities emerge through a rhythmical process of struggling to integrate the unfamiliar with the familiar. In the process of transforming, an individual's diverse patterns arise through integrating new discoveries while continuously becoming the not-yet. Threads of consistency are apparent in the process of integrating, specifying the all-at-once presence of who one is, was, and will become. This all-at-once presence is the unitary cocreated process that is the unique human's pattern. The individual is recognized through this pattern that incarnates chosen values in a coherent connectedness of the familiar-unfamiliar. Dilthey (1961) reflects on this when he says, "The person who seeks the connecting threads in the history of his life has already, from different points of view, created a coherence in that life . . . by experiencing values and realizing purposes" (p. 86). In the process of transforming, then, the human experiences struggling and leaping beyond in continuous movement with diversity.

The ongoing process of change has been described by Watzlawick, Weakland, and Fisch (1974) in a two-level framework as first-order and second-order change. First-order change occurs within the system itself without changing the structure of that system. Types of first-order change are exception, increment, and pendulum shift. Second-order change occurs in the structure of the system itself. It is a whole pattern change, a transforming of the nature of the system.

Consistent with Watzlawick et al.'s (1974) definition of second-order change is Ferguson's (1980) definition of transforming as the "fourth dimension of change: the new perspective, the insight that allows the information to come together in a new form or structure" (p. 72). It is a deliberate shift in one's way of viewing the familiar. The human is available to go with the possibilities of transforming or shifting views in the process of discovering the new in situation. Personal meanings emerge in the human-universe process as individuals view themselves, as well as view themselves being viewed by others. One's view of the other's view is a metaperspective (Laing, Phillipson, & Lee, 1966). These various perspectives emerge with the discovering and creating of possibilities in transforming. As one experiences these perspectives in the gaze, dialogue, and touch of others, the realization of what one envisions one is not all-at-once emerges with what one envisions one is and can become. Discovering perspectives that were previously present only in prereflective awareness calls one to a different and unfamiliar way of viewing the familiar, the creating of a different meaning of a situation. Creating a different meaning is changing the conceptual viewpoint relative to a situation, that is, placing it in another light that fits the facts of the same situation, thereby changing its entire meaning (Watzlawick et al., 1974). The meaning changes as the different perspectives shed new light on the situation, much like the changing reflections as light shines through a prism. New light is shed as a burst of insight illuminates the situation from a different vantage point (Ferguson, 1980). The move to a different vantage point is a shift in one's changing worldview, a changing of change. This changing of change is transforming, deliberately choosing a new view and, in so doing, a new way of becoming. The human's continuous transforming is a personal creative endeavor. When one has chosen a shift to a new insight, one cannot return to viewing the situation in the old way but can only move with other possibles.

For example, the Evans family (Mr. and Mrs. Evans and three teenage children, Barry, Patty, and Lucy) exemplifies transforming as it relates to human becoming. Mr. Evans consults with the family, but is generally responsible for major family decisions. This is the Evans family pattern of decision making. Mrs. Evans' mother, Mrs. Olds, is 76 and self-sufficient. Recently, she has been complaining of a lack of energy. After a complete medical examination, the physician made no specific diagnosis for the "draggy feeling with no pep" that Mrs. Olds expressed frequently. The family talked with Mrs. Olds about her apparent lack of enthusiasm for life, lack of desire to cook for herself and maintain a residence, and apparent search for a reason to live. The Evans family discussed the possibilities for Mrs. Olds, one of which was to invite her to live with them. All the members of the Evans family agreed that Mrs. Olds wanted to be needed and to have a purpose in life. The option to have Mrs. Olds move in with the Evans family was viewed by Mr. Evans, Barry, and Lucy as an intrusion on their lifestyle. Barry and Lucy said that it would interfere with parties and other activities in the home. Mr. Evans thought that Mrs. Evans would "tie herself down" if her mother moved into the family home. Mrs. Evans and Patty talked with Mr. Evans, Barry, and Lucy at length about their way of being with the situation. Mrs. Olds had often participated in the Evans family's life in earlier years, especially when the children were young and Mrs. Olds was needed for help. The family members' perspectives of each other surfaced in the discussion and prompted each member to contemplate how he or she was viewed by others in this group, and the decision about Mrs. Olds moving into the Evans home became an important issue for the family. Mr. Evans began seriously to consider his wife's way of looking at him, prompted primarily by the comment that "Mom was 'good old Mom' when we needed her so that I could participate in your business endeavors—I just can't believe you are resisting helping my mother now—I've never known you this way." Mr. Evans saw himself being seen differently by Mrs. Evans. He then saw himself differently. He spoke with the children about the issue. Barry and Lucy said, "Hold your ground, Dad; Grandma's great, but to live with us is another story." The usually quiet Patty winced when she said, "Dad, we have to help Grandma." Mr. Evans saw what Mrs. Evans and the children said he was not and also possibilities of who he could become. He began to consider the perspectives of himself that surfaced in this situation that had not surfaced before. Mr. Evans attended to creating a different meaning in this situation. He had further discussions with Mrs. Evans, and one afternoon he mentioned the situation to a close friend who joined the family for lunch: "We're talking about having my mother-in-law live with us. I don't know about such a move." The friend immediately said, "Oh, you mean Mrs. Olds will be moving in to help manage the household so you and your wife can be free to travel and expand your business. What a help she'll be with your kids. You're lucky." Mr. Evans said, "Well, I hadn't thought about it quite that way." Mr. Evans' view of the friend's view of the situation created a different meaning for him. The other family members also began to consider the situation in a new light, one that focused attention on the asset Mrs. Olds could be to the family. After much discussion on the new meaning, Mrs. Olds was invited to move into the Evans' home to participate in managing the household. In the excitement of moving in with the Evans family, Mrs. Olds' patterns changed. She had a new spark and lightness. She said she was delighted with the opportunity to help manage the Evans household.

The transforming emerged in the engagement of the Evans family members with a friend as their various perspectives surfaced and cocreated the possibility for a new meaning in this situation. The family was available to see a new view of the familiar and the unfamiliar, and the situation was available to be viewed in a new way. The new meaning shifted worldviews, changing the family's way of being with Mrs. Olds' moving into the Evans' family home. Transforming, a concept of cotranscending with the possibles, is a recognizable feature of human becoming.

The three principles just discussed, with their essential concepts, describe human becoming. Human becoming is structuring meaning multidimensionally in cocreating rhythmical patterns of relating while cotranscending with the possibles. It is the day-to-day creating of reality through the languaging of valuing and imaging as the paradoxical rhythmical patterns of revealing-concealing, enabling-limiting, and connecting-separating are powering ways of originating transforming. The human participates with the universe in creating health and quality of life by choosing imaged values in multidimensional experiences that are the human's paradoxical ways of relating. Ways of relating are rhythms lived as the human comes to know explicitly-tacitly, while confirming-not confirming cherished beliefs in speaking-being silent and moving-being still in the struggle of pushing-resisting with the conformity-non-conformity and certainty-uncertainty in inventing unique ways of viewing the familiar-unfamiliar. This is human becoming.

The principles and concepts of human becoming give rise to theoretical structures. A theoretical structure is a statement interrelating concepts in a unique way. Some emergent theoretical structures of human becoming are listed below.

- Theoretical Structure 1: Powering emerges with the revealing-concealing of imaging.
- Theoretical Structure 2: Originating emerges with the enabling-limiting of valuing.
- Theoretical Structure 3: Transforming emerges with the languaging of connecting-separating.

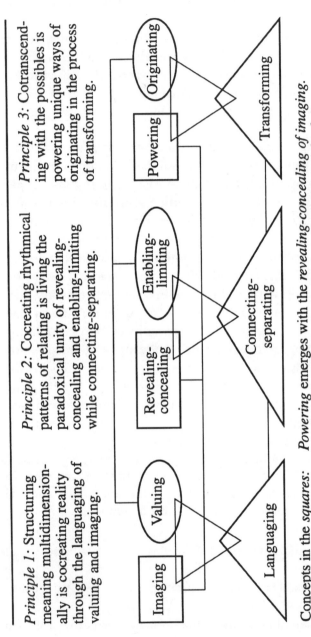

Figure 4.1. Principles, Concepts, and Theoretical Structures of Human Becoming

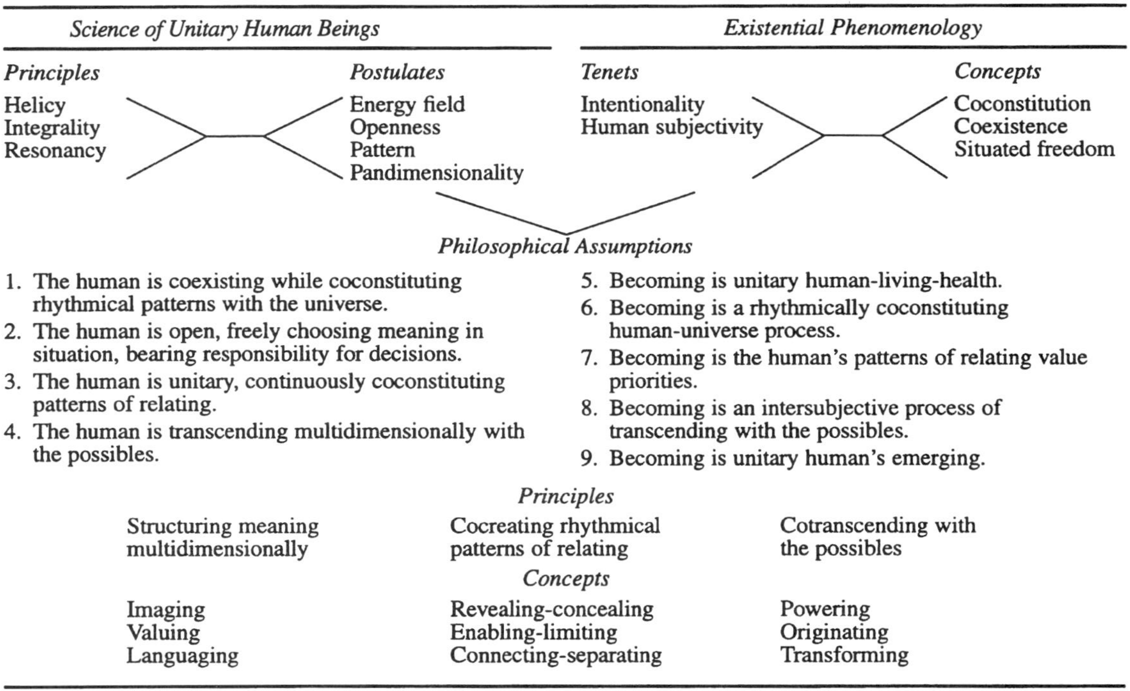

Science of Unitary Human Beings			Existential Phenomenology		
Principles	*Postulates*	*Concepts*	*Tenets*	*Postulates*	*Concepts*
Helicy	Energy field		Intentionality		Coconstitution
Integrality	Openness		Human subjectivity		Coexistence
Resonance	Pattern				Situated freedom
	Pandimensionality				

Philosophical Assumptions

1. The human is coexisting while coconstituting rhythmical patterns with the universe.

5. Becoming is unitary human-living-health.

2. The human is open, freely choosing meaning in situation, bearing responsibility for decisions.

6. Becoming is a rhythmically coconstituting human-universe process.

3. The human is unitary, continuously coconstituting patterns of relating.

7. Becoming is the human's patterns of relating value priorities.

4. The human is transcending multidimensionally with the possibles.

8. Becoming is an intersubjective process of transcending with the possibles.

9. Becoming is unitary human's emerging.

Principles

Structuring meaning multidimensionally

Cocreating rhythmical patterns of relating

Cotranscending with the possibles

Concepts

Imaging
Valuing
Languaging

Revealing-concealing
Enabling-limiting
Connecting-separating

Powering
Originating
Transforming

Figure 4.2. Evolution of the Ontology of Human Becoming

Figure 4.1 shows the emergence of the theoretical structures. Other structures may be generated to guide research and practice. Figure 4.2 depicts the evolution of the ontology of human becoming.

Summary

Human becoming is a school of thought grounded in the human sciences. The ontology consists of the assumptions and principles. The assumptions were synthesized from principles, tenets, postulates, and concepts from the science of unitary human beings and existential phenomenology. The three principles and nine concepts with paradoxes of human becoming follow.

Principle 1: Structuring meaning multidimensionally

Concepts	Paradoxes
Imaging	Reflective-prereflective; explicit-tacit
Valuing	Confirming-not confirming
Languaging	Speaking-being silent; moving-being still

Principle 2: Cocreating rhythmical patterns of relating

Concepts and Paradoxes
Revealing-concealing
Enabling-limiting
Connecting-separating

Principle 3: Cotranscending with the possibles

Concepts	Paradoxes
Powering	Pushing-resisting; affirming-not affirming; being-nonbeing
Originating	Conformity-nonconformity; certainty-uncertainty
Transforming	Familiar-unfamiliar

CHAPTER 5

HUMAN BECOMING IN RESEARCH, PRACTICE, AND EDUCATION

Research, Practice, and Education

The human becoming school of thought consists of the ontology (assumptions and principles) and the epistemology and the methodologies (research and practice). The assumptions and the principles (referred to as the *theory*) of human becoming were discussed in Chapters 3, "Assumptions About the Human and Becoming," and 4, "Principles, Concepts, and Theoretical Structures of Human Becoming." This chapter explicates the research and practice methodologies and specifies some aspects of a curriculum for a master's program.

The interrelationship among theory, research, practice, and education is the foundation of the evolution of nursing as a science and an art. Theory creatively invented from a conceptual system and philosophical assumptions is enhanced through scholarly research. Scholarly research is formal inquiry leading to the discovery of new knowledge with the enhancement of theory. It includes rigorous conceptual, ethical, methodological, and interpretive phases. The conceptual phase includes the description of the phenomenon, the research question, and the frame of reference; the ethical dimension includes the scientific integrity of the research study and protection of participants' rights; the methodological phase includes participant selection, data gathering, and data analysis-synthesis; and the interpretive phase includes the connection of the findings to the frame of reference and other related literature with specific implications for theory development, further research, and practice. Research described in this way does not include problem-solving projects related to nursing practice situations that involve trial-and-error mechanisms or to the systematic inquiry projects that culminate in reviews of literature. These do not lead to new knowledge about phenomena.

The findings of nursing research (formal inquiry) enhance theories and conceptual systems, expanding the body of nursing knowledge. Nursing knowledge is the theoretical base embedded in the nursing frameworks taught in nursing schools; it guides nursing practice. The changing human-universe process spawns new situations for nursing practice, creating new possibilities for research that, when pursued, enhance nursing's knowledge base. Nursing knowledge is the rightful content of nursing curricula. Doctoral curricula, particularly, focus on nursing research, providing educational guidance for those preparing to be leaders in enhancing the knowledge base of nursing. The interrelationship among theory, research, practice, and education is a mutual process significant to the evolution of nursing as a science and an art rooted in its own unique body of knowledge.

Sciencing Human Becoming

Sciencing human becoming is the process of coming to know and understand human experiences. The term *sciencing*, different from science, is used to reflect inquiry as an ongoing process (White, 1938). Since the early 1980s, sciencing human becoming has been through borrowed research methods—descriptive exploratory from the social sciences, phenomenological (van Kaam and Giorgi modifications) from existential phenomenological psychology, and ethnography from anthropology (see Banonis, 1989; Baumann, 1994; Costello-Nickitas, 1994; Davis & Cannava, 1995; Futrell, Wondolowski, & Mitchell, 1993; Jonas, 1992; Mitchell, 1994; Nokes & Carver, 1991; Parse, 1993, 1996b; Parse et al., 1985; Rendon, Sales, Leal, & Pique, 1995; Wondolowski & Davis, 1991). These studies all add to the knowledge base of nursing and expanded understanding of the phenomena under study.

Since the mid-1980s, there have been two types of research studies (see Table 5.1) specifically related to the human becoming school of thought and unique to sciencing in nursing. One type is *basic* research, which may be conducted with the goal of uncovering the structure of lived experiences to expand knowledge of the science (Parse, 1987, 1990b, 1995, 1996a, 1997a, 1997b), or may be an interpretative hermeneutic process that specifies the meaning of texts from the human becoming perspective (Cody, 1995b). The other type is *applied* research, the goal of which is to evaluate human becoming as a guide to practice. The findings of this type of research do not enhance the knowledge base of the theory per se, but they do show what happens when human becoming guides practice in various settings (Parse, 1995).

Human Becoming Basic Research

The Parse Research Methodology

The Parse research methodology was constructed in congruence with the principles of human becoming (Parse, 1981, 1987, 1990b, 1992, 1995, 1997a, 1997b). The principles of methodology construction (Parse, 1987, p. 173) follow.

1. The methodology is constructed to be in harmony with and evolve from the ontological beliefs of the research tradition.
2. The methodology is an overall design of precise processes that adhere to scientific rigor.
3. The methodology specifies the order within the processes appropriate for inquiry within the research tradition.

TABLE 5.1 Human Becoming Methods of Inquiry

	Basic Research	Applied Research
Purpose	To advance the science of human becoming	To evaluate the changes and effectiveness of health care when the human becoming theory guides practice
Methods	Parse Method	Descriptive Qualitative Preproject-Process-Postproject Method
	Human Becoming Hermeneutic Method	
Phenomena	Lived experiences (descriptions from participants)	Change, satisfaction, and effectiveness (descriptions from participants and documents)
	Lived experiences (descriptions from published texts)	
Processes	Dialogical engagement	Preproject information gathering by evaluator
	Extraction-synthesis	Teaching-learning sessions on human becoming theory in practice
	Heuristic interpretation	Midway information gathering by evaluator
	Discoursing	Teaching-learning sessions (continued)
	Interpreting	Postproject information gathering by evaluator
	Understanding	Analysis-synthesis of themes from each information source
		Synthesis of themes from all information sources
Discover	The paradoxical living of the remembered, the now moment, and the not-yet all-at-once	Thematic conceptualizations
	Emergent meanings	
Contributions	New knowledge and understanding of humanly lived experiences to guide further research and practice	Knowledge about the changes in, satisfaction with, and effectiveness of health care when the human becoming theory guides practice to expand ways to initiate and fortify this theory as a basis for practice in a variety of settings

62

4. The methodology is an aesthetic composition with balance in form.

The basic assumptions (Parse, 1992, p. 41) underlying the Parse method follow.

1. Humans are open beings in mutual process with the universe. The construct *human becoming* refers to the human-universe-health process.
2. Human becoming is uniquely lived by individuals. People make reflective-prereflective choices in connection with others and the universe that incarnate their health.
3. Descriptions of lived experiences enhance knowledge of human becoming. Individuals and families can describe their own experiences in ways that shed light on the meaning of health.
4. Researcher-participant dialogical engagement uncovers the meaning of phenomena as humanly lived. The researcher in true presence with the participant can elicit authentic information about lived experiences.
5. The researcher, through inventing, abiding with logic, and adhering to semantic consistency during the extraction-synthesis and heuristic interpretation processes, creates structures of lived experiences and weaves the structure with the theory in ways that enhance the knowledge base of nursing.

The research method, somewhat different from other qualitative methods (Giorgi, 1970, 1971, 1985; Spiegelberg, 1976), is a phenomenological-hermeneutic method in that the universal experiences described by participants who lived them provide the source of information, and participants' descriptions are interpreted in light of the human becoming theory (see Table 5.2). The phenomena for study are universal lived experiences of health, such as hope, joy-sorrow, contentment, grieving, and suffering. Participants are persons who can describe the meaning of the experience under study through words, symbols, music, metaphors, poetry, photographs, drawings, or movements.

The processes of the method follow.

TABLE 5.2 Differences Between the Parse Method and Similar
Qualitative Research Methods

Research Dimensions	Parse Method	Similar Qualitative Methods
Conceptual	Phenomena for study are universal human health experiences.	Phenomena may be lived experiences.
Ethical	Scientific integrity is preserved, and participants' rights are protected.	Scientific integrity is preserved, and rights of participants are protected.
Methodological	Dialogical engagement is a researcher-participant dialogue that elicits descriptions. It is true presence, not an interview.	Retrospective descriptions, participant observation, and structured and unstructured interviews are used to elicit descriptions from participants.
	Extraction-synthesis moves participants' descriptions to synthesized structures of lived experiences.	Analysis-synthesis moves data from concrete descriptions to themes.
Interpretive	Heuristic interpretation weaves the structure with the human becoming theory and beyond through structural transposition and conceptual integration to enhance understanding of phenomena and expand knowledge about human experiences.	Conclusions are drawn and hypotheses are generated through logical abstraction, sometimes to provide a basis for quantitative research.

1. *Dialogical engagement* is not an interview but, rather, a discussion between the researcher and participant, in true presence, that focuses on the phenomenon under study as it is described by the participant. These dialogues are audiotaped and, when possible, videotaped. The researcher centers prior to the engagement with each participant and, after the appropriate consent for protection of participants is signed, opens the dialogue with a comment such as, "Please tell me about your experience of . . ." The researcher enters the flow with each

participant as the participant relates a description about the phenomenon under study. The researcher stays in true presence with the participant without interjecting questions, but may move the discussion by saying something such as, "Go on" or "Please explain more about your experience of . . ."

2. *Extraction-synthesis* is culling the essences from the dialogue in the language of the participant and conceptualizing these essences in the language of science to form a structure of the experience. This process occurs through dwelling with the transcribed audiotaped and videotaped dialogues in deep concentration to elicit the meaning of the experience as described by participants, inventing through abiding with logic, and adhering to semantic consistency. The structure (the paradoxical living of the remembered, the now moment, and the not-yet all-at-once) arising from this process is the answer to the research question. The process follows:

a. Extracting and synthesizing essences from transcribed and recorded descriptions in the participant's language
b. Synthesizing and extracting essences in the researcher's language
c. Formulating a proposition from each participant's essences
d. Extracting and synthesizing core concepts from the formulated propositions of all participants
e. Synthesizing a structure of the lived experience from the core concepts

3. *Heuristic interpretation* weaves the structure with the principles of human becoming and beyond to enhance the knowledge base and create ideas for further research (Parse, 1987, 1992, 1995, 1997a). Structural transposition and conceptual integration are the processes of heuristic interpretation that move the discourse of the structure to the discourse of the theory (for further details regarding the method, see Parse, 1987, 1990b, 1992, 1995, 1997a, 1997b). The findings from studies conducted using the Parse methodology contributed new knowledge and understanding of human experiences, adding to the knowledge base

of nursing on phenomena such as going along when one does
not believe (Kelley, 1991), grieving (Cody, 1991, 1995a; Pilkington, 1993), hope (Parse, 1990b; Thornburg, 1993; Wang, 1997),
taking life day by day (Mitchell, 1990), struggling through a
difficult time (Smith, 1990), considering tomorrow (Bunkers, in
press), persevering through a difficult time (Petardi, in press),
feeling alone while with others (Gouty, 1996), suffering (Daly,
1995), laughing and health (Parse, 1994b), joy-sorrow (Parse,
1997b), and many others.

The Human Becoming Hermeneutic Method

Hermeneutics is a mode of inquiry that focuses on *interpretation* and *understanding*. It is a dialogical process between researcher and text uncovering meaning interpreted through a
particular perspective. The interpretation itself is the meaning
given to the text from the frame of reference of the researcher;
thus, the understanding of the text incarnates that frame of reference. Dilthey (1961, 1976, 1883/1988) first posited hermeneutics
as a mode of inquiry for the human sciences when he proposed
interpretation as significant for the study of all human projects
(Dilthey, 1883/1988; Ermarth, 1978; Polkinghorne, 1983).
Heidegger (1962) sets forth the idea that there is ontological
grounding with hermeneutics, and Gadamer (1975, 1976) elaborates this notion when he describes the idea of "fusion of horizons" as what arises "when the text and interpreter meet in
dialogue" (Parse, 1996a, p. 12). From the human becoming perspective, Cody (1995b) identifies three processes of hermeneutics: discoursing, interpreting, and understanding. These are the
processes lived in the researcher-text dialogue. In general with
hermeneutics, it is important for the researcher to specify the
frame of reference with which she or he approaches the text so
that the emergent meanings uncovered in the interpretation can
be understood by the reader (Parse, 1995, 1996a). For example,
if a researcher chooses to conduct a hermeneutic study of a
literary work or other text from the human becoming perspective, the interpretation will emerge in the language of the principles of human becoming (see Cody, 1995b). The interpretation

in this case adds knowledge to nursing about lived experiences from a human becoming perspective.

Human Becoming Applied Research

An applied research method, the preproject-process-postproject descriptive qualitative method that is compatible with the principles of human becoming, is appropriate for evaluating the theory in practice. The purpose of the method is to ascertain specific changes that emerge after initiation of the human becoming theory in practice. The information is gathered prior to the initiation of the project, midway, and at the end of the project. Information sources include direct observation of nurses' documentation; written and tape-recorded interviews with nurses regarding their beliefs about human beings, health, and nursing; tape-recorded interviews with persons and their families regarding their experiences with nursing care; and tape-recorded interviews with nurse managers, physicians, and other multidisciplinary health care providers. An evaluator who is not engaged in the day-to-day activity of the setting makes a record of the responses from the information sources before the teaching-learning process sessions on human becoming commence, midway through the study, and at the end of the project. The teaching-learning process takes place on a regular basis within the time frame of the study. A human becoming nurse specialist instructs study participants (nurses and other health care providers) about the theory and guides them in consistent practice and documentation after preproject information gathering is completed. Practice consistent with the human becoming theory follows the practice methodology of illuminating meaning, synchronizing rhythms, and mobilizing transcendence (Parse, 1987, 1992, 1995, 1997a). The study participants learn the methodology, along with the basic beliefs set forth in the human becoming school of thought. They learn that living the theory shows itself in true presence with others.

Committing to practice from a human becoming perspective is a paradigm shift, takes concentrated study over time, and is reflected in the care with and documentation about those receiving service. In settings where formal documentation is required, a personal health description; patterns of becoming; nurse-person activities; and plans, goals, and priorities for change are included in an easy-to-access format that can be determined by nurses. *Personal health descriptions* include the meanings of the situation, the relationship with close others, and the hopes and wishes articulated by the recipient of care. *Patterns of becoming* are themes surfacing in discussion, are paradoxical, and guide nurse-person activities. *Nurse-person activities* are those in which the nurse participates as decided by the recipient of care. *Plans, goals, and priorities for change* in personal patterns of becoming are written from the perspective of the recipient of care. Changing patterns are described by the person and may be recorded by the nurse or the person (Parse, 1989). After the end-of-project information gathering is completed, each set of descriptions is analyzed and synthesized to arrive at themes from each source. These themes are further synthesized to answer the research question: What changes emerge in nurses' beliefs and practice, persons' and families' experiences of health care, and opinions of multidisciplinary health care providers when the human becoming theory is initiated as a guide to practice? Thematic conceptualizations arise from this synthesis.

Findings from these studies add knowledge and understanding about the effectiveness of the human becoming theory in practice, and are valuable for changing health care patterns. All the published studies have shown that the human becoming theory in practice was effective and led to major changes in nurses' beliefs about people and health care practices, changes in persons' and families' satisfaction with health care, and changes in opinions about nursing from multidisciplinary health care providers (see Jonas, 1995; Mitchell, 1995; Northrup & Cody, in press; Santopinto & Smith, 1995).

Living the Art of Human Becoming

The art of living human becoming is guided by the theoretical principles that espouse the human as free agent and meaning-giver, choosing rhythmical patterns of relating while reaching for personal hopes and dreams. The art of nursing is using nursing's abstract body of knowledge in service to people. The contexts in which nursing arises are nurse-person and nurse-group situations. Nursing takes place with children and adults, in homes, shelters, health care centers, parish halls, all departments of hospitals or clinics, rehabilitation centers, offices, and other milieus where nurses are with people. The goal of the discipline of nursing is quality of life from the person's, family's, and community's perspective. The human becoming nurse's goal is to be truly present with people as they enhance their quality of life. "Quality of life as the incarnation of lived experiences is the indivisible human's view on living moment to moment as the changing patterns of shifting perspectives weave the fabric of life through the human-universe interconnectedness" (Parse, 1994c, p. 17). Quality of life can be described only by the person or persons living the life, because it is the incarnation of meanings in their seamless symphony of becoming. Quality or whatness is the essence of something—in this case, the essence of life, the core substance that makes a life different and uniquely irreplaceable. The nurse living human becoming "respects each individual's or family's own view of quality and does not attempt to change that view to be consistent with his or her own perspective" (Parse, 1992, p. 39).

The Human Becoming Practice Methodology

From the perspective of the human becoming school of thought in focusing on quality of life, the nurse is guided to be in true presence in living the dimensions and processes of the practice methodology that were designed in congruence with the principles (Parse, 1987, 1992, 1995, 1997a). These dimensions and processes follow.

1. Illuminating meaning is explicating what was, is, and will be. *Explicating* is making clear what is appearing now through languaging.

2. Synchronizing rhythms is dwelling with the pitch, yaw, and roll of the human-universe process. *Dwelling with* is immersing with the flow of connecting-separating.
3. Mobilizing transcendence is moving beyond the meaning moment with what is not-yet. *Moving beyond* is propelling with envisioned possibles of transforming (Parse, 1987, 1992, 1995, 1997a).

The nurse, with the person, family, or community, invites a discussion of the meaning of the situation. In telling about the meaning, persons share thoughts and feelings with themselves, the nurse, and others in nurse-family-community situations. The process of explicating sheds a new light on situations, and often the thoughts and feelings discussed have been lying dormant beneath the surface for some time. Articulation of such thoughts connected with the moment in the presence of the nurse may surface with *ah-has*, which are ways of viewing the familiar in a new light. The nurse stays with persons as they describe the ups and downs, struggles, moments of joy, and the unevenness of day-to-day living in the now moment. The nurse living the human becoming theory does not try to calm uneven rhythms but, rather, goes with the rhythms set by the person, family, or community. The nurse moves with the flow of the rhythms as persons discuss and recognize the ups and downs, joys and sorrows within the struggles of the situation (Parse, 1987, 1992, 1995, 1997a). Dwelling with the rhythms or staying with the flow is like treading water: While one appears to remain in the same place, different waves arise to create subtle movements or gigantic leaps. Persons, families, and community groups move beyond the moment, reaching the hopes and dreams that have been illuminated through the process of being with the nurse. The hopes are anticipations of what is desired and the dreams are imaginings that arise at various realms of the universe, immersing the person or group with possibles yet-to-be. The moving beyond arises as the rhythmical dwelling of nurse with person, family, or group erupts in explications of the situation that incarnate new meanings. The human becoming

nurse lives true presence with others in the processes of illuminating meaning, synchronizing rhythms, and mobilizing transcendence.

True Presence

True presence is a special way of "being with" in which the
nurse is attentive to moment-to-moment changes in meaning as
she or he bears witness to the person's or group's own living of
value priorities. True presence is an intentional reflective love,
an interpersonal art grounded in a strong knowledge base,

> reflecting the belief that each person knows "the way" somewhere
> within self. Each human lives a way, his or her *own* way, which is
> both alike and different from the "ways" of others. It is *like* that of
> others in that it is a personal way of being. It is *different* from others
> in that it is one's own. It is like a fingerprint in that it belongs to
> only one human being and while others coexist in the large journey
> of life, each lives his or her own way on the journey. (Parse, 1990a,
> p. 139)

True presence is a powerful human-universe connection experienced at all realms of the universe. It is being with the
rhythms of the sounds and silences, the visions and blindnesses
of the human-universe process. True presence is a free-flowing
attentiveness that does not arise from trying to attend to the
other, because the *trying to* is a distraction that demands a focus
away from the other. To be with another or a group in the
free-flowing active stillness of true presence, preparation and
attention are essential. *Preparation* involves an emptying to be
available to bear witness to the other or others. To be available
to bear witness is being flexible, not fixed but gracefully present
from one's center. The nurse prepares through dwelling with the
universe at the moment, considering the attentive presence
about to be. *Attention* is focus. To attend to is to focus on the
moment at hand for immersion. Immersion with the intent of
true presence cocreates attentiveness to the other (Parse, 1994c).

Thus, true presence already begins in the coming-to-be-present moments of preparation and attention prior to coming together with the other or others. The *coming-to-be-present* through preparation and attention is an all-at-once gentling down and lifting up. It is taking a stand, an unencumbered soft foothold in a tranquil flow, a gentle ease and quiet slowness that moves the nurse and person or group to the tacit-explicit knowing of the messages given and taken at many realms of the universe. The rhythmical patterns arising in the coming together shed light on meaning and moving beyond (Parse, 1997a).

The nurse enters the person's or group's world as a not-knowing stranger (Parse, 1996c). The person's or group's world is a personal reality, the history of lived moments known only to the person or group explicitly-tacitly. Persons share with the nurse only the reality that they wish to disclose. The nurse in true presence joins the reality of others at all realms of the universe and is available to bear witness without judging or labeling. Persons at all realms of the universe experience the intent of the nurse, which is to bear witness to changing health patterns. The intent of the nurse is languaged in his or her whole being, in the subtle knowings of the messages given and taken at all realms of the universe, so words are not necessary to live true presence in the nurse-person or nurse-group process. The nurse is with the other(s) in true presence through face-to-face discussions, silent immersions, and lingering presence (Parse, 1997a).

Face-to-Face Discussions

In face-to-face discussions, the nurse and person or group engage in dialogue. The conversation may be through discussion in general or through interpretations of stories, films, drawings, photographs, music, metaphors, poetry, rhythmic movements, and other expressions. For example, persons have expressed their thoughts of health by drawing pictures, such as a rainbow or a bubbling brook. Some have selected photographs of friends and strangers in various settings that represented their thoughts of the moment on their health, and others have written stories or poetry about lost loved ones to describe their grieving or participated in writing songs about the meaning of their experiences. Some groups have watched films together and discussed these in light of their situations. All nurse-person or nurse-group processes, through whatever medium, are led by the person or group.

Silent Immersion

Silent immersion is a process of the quiet that does not refrain from sending and receiving messages. It is a deep place of no words that symbolizes much, a soundless hush of wordless stillness that arises in a moment of cocreating with others, ideas, objects, and situations. Silent immersion is a chosen way of becoming in the human-universe process lived in the rhythm of speaking-being silent, moving-being still, as valued images incarnate meaning. Silent immersion is true presence without words, just "being with" through immediate engaging in the presence of another or through imagination with a grounding in the intention to bear witness to the other's becoming. The intention is felt and disclosed at many realms of the universe as the nurse embraces the other (or others) as knowing his or her way (Parse, 1994c, 1997a). Honoring the other is known in the messages given and taken as nurse and person(s) live with the multidimensional realities of their moments together and apart.

Lingering Presence

Living the remembered is recalling a moment through a lingering presence that arises after an immediate engagement, "a reflective-prereflective 'abiding with' attended to through glimpses of the other person, idea, object, or situation" (Parse, 1994c, p. 19). The glimpses may surface "moments, days, or years later—and they can be startling surprises, calming excursions, or uncomfortable intrusions" (Parse, 1994c, p. 19). The true presence is inextricably woven into the fabric of one's life, whether it is explicitly remembered or not.

Ways of Changing Health in True Presence

People may change health patterns in true presence with the nurse when they change their value priorities, since health is a personal commitment cocreated with others (Parse, 1981, 1990a, 1992). Some ways one moves through moments in changing health include creative imagining, affirming personal becoming, and glimpsing the paradoxical. Through *creative imagining*, one can picture—that is, see, hear, and feel—what a situation might be like if lived in a different way. Imagining is structuring a scenario in which a change is already made, trying it on, getting a feel for it, seeing what a change might be like through anticipatory projecting; for example, structuring a scenario around what a move to a different job would be like, or different living arrangements, or walking erect if one has been immobile. Creative imagining, when seriously approached as a way of moving with the moment, immerses the person with the structured situation. This profound immersion is a way of experiencing a change and learning about what might be while evolving with the imaged possibles. The notion was shown in the findings from a study by Parse (1990b) on hope using the Parse research methodology with 10 participants on hemodialysis. The structure is "hope is anticipating possibilities through envisioning the not-yet in harmoniously living the comfort-discomfort of everydayness while unfolding a different perspective of an expanding view" (p. 15). In dialogical engagement with the researcher, participants shared that persistent picturing of possibles, such as having a kidney transplant, seeing a daughter graduate from college, and traveling to another county to visit family, moved them beyond the moment and changed their experience of health. The persistent picturing of something that was not-yet moved these persons to another experience. LeShan (1982) believes that if you believe it, you will be it! Creative imagining is persistent picturing of something that is not-yet, and is a way of changing meaning, thus changing the personal commitment that is health.

Affirming personal becoming is another way of moving beyond the moment. Affirming is explicitly-tacitly living patterns that incarnate the who one is becoming. In critically thinking about

how or who one is, one uncovers personal patterns of preference. These patterns of preference affirm becoming a certain
way. To persist in living these patterns of preference confirms
the specific values by which a person is known. For example, a
person who believes he or she is unhappy will live a set of values
that perpetuates this belief. To change living unhappy to happy
living, new persistent patterns consistent with happy are will-
fully created. The "I will" and "I can" attitude toward a given
desire for change creates it and affirms a different way, thus
changing health.

Glimpsing the paradoxical in changing health is looking at the
incongruence in a situation as the apparent opposites inevitably
surface. The recognition of incongruence sheds a different light
on an apparent conflict and changes the view of something.
From a phenomenological study by Parse (1993) in which 30
persons over 65 were asked to describe a situation in which they
experienced laughing their heart out, the structural description
emerged as "laughing is a buoyant immersion in the presence
of unanticipated glimpsings prompting harmonious integrity
which surfaces anew in contemplative visioning" (p. 41). Participants in this study said that laughter arose when they viewed
a difficult situation in a different light, and this changed their
way of living the moment.

Glimpsing the paradoxical, whether prompting laughter or
not, is a way of moving beyond the moment in changing patterns of health. For example, persons who glimpse some of the
incongruities of serious situations may change their views of the
situations. This moves them beyond the moment and changes
the emerging patterns of health.

Creative imagining, affirming personal becoming, and
glimpsing the paradoxical are ways that can move persons
beyond to change patterns of health. These ways of changing
health patterns arise in the true presence of the nurse. The nurse
in true presence with a person or group, then, is not a guide or
a beacon, but an inspiring attentive presence that calls others to
shed light on the meaning moments of life, bearing witness to
the choices in changing health patterns. It is the person, family,
or group in the presence of the nurse who illuminates the

meaning, synchronizes the rhythms, and mobilizes transcendence in moving beyond. Persons coauthor health, as free agents and meaning givers, choosing rhythmical patterns of relating while reaching for personal hopes and dreams.

For nursing practice, being in true presence with another means that all realms of the universe of the nurse and the person(s) are interconnecting, reflectively-prereflectively; thus, how the nurse is with the person(s) is extremely important since multiple messages are both given and taken and somehow live on with both. True presence, nurse with person or group, then, is a human-universe cocreation of becoming. This way of being present is valuing the others' human dignity and freedom to choose within situations, and it is fundamental to living the art of human becoming, the focus of which is the quality of life from the person's or group's perspective.

Family Situation:
An Example

An example of a family situation follows, with a discussion related to the theory of human becoming. The description of the family, the decision-making pattern, and the family's contextual situation emerged in several meetings between the family and the nurse. The nurse was in true presence with the family as the members illuminated meaning, synchronized rhythms, and mobilized transcendence in their changing health patterns.

Descriptions of Family Members

Mr. and Mrs. Taylor have two children: Randy, age 18, and Jamie, age 14. From his perspective, Mr. Taylor believes he is ultraconservative and frugal. He says he has a traditional belief system. For example, he believes that women are fragile, weak, and need a man's protection, and that children must honor and obey their parents. He works hard as a comptroller for a large corporation and is the family breadwinner. Mrs. Taylor says Mr. Taylor is her best friend. She says he is strong and provides well for the family but could be more flexible, especially with the children. Randy thinks his father is strict but fair, and says he is sometimes difficult to talk with but would like to be like him. Jamie says her father is kind, hard working, a real protector, easy to get along with, and very strong.

Mrs. Taylor says she is basically conservative, sharing traditional values with her husband, and she tries to live the ideals of a perfect family. She is interested in finding a job outside the home to keep occupied now that the children are grown. Mr. Taylor says his wife is very well organized, a smart household manager, and a good mother. He is proud of her, and stated that she helps everyone. Randy says his mother is gentle, easy to talk to, and understanding. Jamie says her mother is loving, helpful, and very generous.

Randy sees himself as athletic and fun loving. He wants to become an engineer, and says he really likes college life. Mr. Taylor says Randy is a good student and will turn out to be something if he continues to work hard. Mrs. Taylor says Randy is bright, has his "own mind" about things, and is quite opinionated. Jamie thinks her brother is easy to talk to and very considerate. He makes her laugh and helps her with math.

Jamie says she is shy and is not growing up fast enough. She loves singing in the church choir and drawing pictures of nature. Mr. Taylor says Jamie is serious, a good student, and quite pretty. Mrs. Taylor believes that Jamie is quiet, neat, and intelligent. Randy says he loves his sister, and finds her thoughtful and pleasant. He says she is talented, and he appreciates her drawings.

Decision-Making Pattern in the Taylor Family

Mr. and Mrs. Taylor discuss issues and come to mutual agreement on major decisions. The children are becoming more and more a part of the family decision-making process. For example, recently the Taylors decided to purchase an automobile, and all the family members participated in deciding on the model and color.

Contextual Situation

As Mr. Taylor approached his doctor's office, he was annoyed and impatient as he thought about the work waiting for him at his office and the wasted time involved in this annual physical examination. He mused how his wife was much too concerned about these things, and so organized that the visit was planned months ago. In Dr. Brown's office, however, his musing changed.

Mr. Taylor's chest X-ray showed a shadow that could be a tumor, and perhaps a malignant one. Dr. Brown advised Mr. Taylor to have more definitive studies done at once. As Mr. Taylor left the doctor's office, a nurse living the human becoming principles approached him. She introduced herself, and then sat with him and talked about his situation. Mr. Taylor became acutely aware of the potential meanings of the menacing spot; and, as this awareness unfolded for him, new insights and new values surfaced as he dwelled with the remembered and the imaged all-at-once. The nurse listened attentively as he spoke of his wife and children as he confronted the possibilities on how he would share with his family the information about the shadow on his lung. The nurse asked him to imagine telling them in different ways, and he structured scenarios to get comfortable, no longer in a hurry to get back to his office. Mr. Taylor sat on a bench with the nurse outside the medical complex and, for the first time in a long time, said he knew the sunshine on his face and the mild breeze through his hair, and he spoke of these to the nurse. As Mr. Taylor dwelled with one phenomenon after the other in his unfocused imaging in the presence of the nurse, he connected and separated all-at-once multidimensionally. He decided to go home and discuss the matter with Mrs. Taylor before the children arrived home for dinner. The nurse accompanied Mr. Taylor at his request.

In sharing the news with Mrs. Taylor, Mr. Taylor languaged his pain as he sat slumped in the kitchen chair, unable to drink the cup of tea he had requested. The two looked at each other knowingly—both seeing in the other the suffering. In coconstitution with each other, each imaged possibilities. They came to

know, in a new way, their affection for each other and the
children through the surfacing of the potentials of nonbeing, the
not-yet known. The prized values of future planning—a well-
organized household and strict rules—were viewed now with a
different perspective as Mr. and Mrs. Taylor, in the presence of
the nurse, revealed and concealed their hopes and desires, fears
and pain through their gestures, facial expressions, speech, and
silences. As they began to discuss the possibilities in the immediate and long-range future, they uncovered the enabling and
limiting aspects of the event, as they struggled to integrate the
unfamiliar with the familiar. The ambiguity of the situation
permeated the thoughts of Mr. and Mrs. Taylor as they struggled
to be more comfortable with the situation and more certain about
the future. They talked with the nurse about the various meanings
of the situation. They decided to talk with the children about the
situation and share their concerns and the possibilities.

On hearing the news, Jamie cried and hugged Mr. Taylor. She
said she was afraid. Her view of Mr. Taylor as protector was
brought into question as she confronted the meaning of nonbeing for herself and for her father. Randy was quiet, not light-
hearted, as he was confronted with the meaning of the event for
him as the oldest child. He saw his father differently; for the first
time, he saw him as vulnerable, and this surfaced the potential
of nonbeing for him. The Taylor family drew close together in
struggling to transcend with the paradoxes and to create possibilities as the changing health priorities brought other view-
points to the surface. The nurse stayed with the family for
several hours on a number of occasions, bearing witness to the
changing health patterns.

Discussion of Nursing Practice
With the Taylor Family

The nurse was in true presence with the Taylor family, bearing
witness as they illuminated the meaning of their changing situation through words and silences, explicating envisioned possibles. Various perspectives were shared by the family members,

bringing to light new ways to view the familiar and unfamiliar all-at-once. All members disclosed and hid all-at-once their ideas about what this situation of Mr. Taylor's lung spot would mean. The pushing-resisting process rose in the family struggle to clarify the situation, while synchronizing the members' rhythms as attention moved to the possibilities of life not being the same. The nurse invited the family members to imagine the possibilities, and she stayed with their rhythms as they moved beyond the moment, affirming their connecting through creative imagining.

The nurse spoke with the family members about their cherished beliefs as the uncertainty of the situation brought to light the opportunities and restrictions emerging with the changing health patterns. The members shared the meaning of the changing rhythms as they mobilized to create new ways of living with changing value priorities. The family members moved together and apart in synchronizing rhythms and moving beyond with changed meanings.

The new discoveries that surface in nursing practice as the nurse is in true presence with families arise through illuminating meaning, synchronizing rhythms, and mobilizing transcendence.

Education and Human Becoming

Nursing curricula reflect current trends related to nursing's abstract body of knowledge. The purpose of nursing education programs is to transmit the body of nursing knowledge to those who will practice, teach, and conduct research in nursing. The curricula of all programs should reflect this purpose. Doctoral programs in nursing, for example, focus on using and expanding research methodologies, analyzing extant nursing theories, and developing nursing theory to prepare students to design and conduct research studies that will enhance nursing knowledge. A curriculum consistent with the theoretical foundation of human becoming is designed with a deliberate focus on the assumptions, principles, and methodologies of this school of thought. First, emphasis is placed on the philosophy of the program, and this philosophy is present thematically throughout the structure of the curriculum. The principles of human becoming are evident in all the elements of the sample curriculum suggested here: philosophy, program goals, program indicators, conceptual framework, themes, course culture content, instructional strategies, and evaluation strategies.

General Elements of a Curriculum Plan

Program Philosophy and Goals

The *philosophy* of a school of nursing is a comprehensive statement of beliefs representing the collective view of the entire faculty about the human-universe-health process in the scientific discipline of nursing. The statement of beliefs is arrived at through the ongoing process of negotiation as faculty members from diverse educational, social, and philosophical backgrounds come to an agreement on the basic underpinnings and unifying focus of a particular program. All other elements of the curriculum flow from the philosophy.

A philosophy includes a statement of specific beliefs about the human, health, society, education, nursing's emerging role in society, and the teaching-learning process. These beliefs should reflect the general beliefs of the institution of which the school of nursing is a part. The program *goals* are broad aims that clearly reflect the intent of the program; they serve also to guide the faculty, students, and administration in the educational process.

Conceptual framework and themes

A *conceptual framework*, along with its support theories, flows clearly and directly from the philosophy and is the basic architectural blueprint from which the curriculum themes emerge; these themes, then, form the course culture content. The conceptual framework consists of the concepts that surface in the philosophy. The support theories are selected for their consistency with the beliefs outlined in the philosophy, and they complement the nursing theoretical base. The curriculum *themes* are the recurrent and ongoing patterns of ideas that unify all the courses within each level, and all the courses from level to level.

Indicators

Program indicators, when properly constructed, flow from the goals and framework and specifically guide the teaching-learning process. Indicators, like objectives, are beacons on which sights can be set in relation to goal achievement. Unlike objectives, however, indicators are far more general. Although indicators always state specific content and action, they do not identify exactly how a student must perform to achieve a goal. The term *indicator* as used here is a far less specific term than *objective,* and explicitly reflects the subjective nature of all evaluative measures.

Indicators strongly imply the responsibility of both the teacher and the learner in the evaluative process. They allow for deviation from the often abused and historically perpetuated myth that performance can be measured "objectively" by the teacher. When the philosophy of a school of nursing espouses the notion that evaluation of students is a cocreated process, teacher with student, the term *indicator* should be used instead of the term *objective* to promote and foster internal congruence in the overall curriculum design. Indicator, then, is used in the design of a comprehensive curriculum plan whose theoretical underpinnings are based on a belief about the human as an open being cocreating a personal becoming. *Level indicators* flow from the program goals and indicators. The level indicators identify the expected achievement in performance after the student has accrued a certain number of credit hours in a particular program. Each set of level indicators refers directly to a particular program goal and gives rise to the course goals and the indicators taught within that particular level. The course goals and indicators are the specific guides for student achievement in an individual course. The goals guide and focus the development of the course culture content. A synthesis of the course goals and indicators at a given level, then, are that level's indicators.

Course Culture Content

Course culture content refers to the specific conceptual focus of each separate unit of instruction. It reflects the conceptual framework, its support theories, and the entirety of its unifying themes, thus reflecting the philosophy of the program.

Evaluation Process

The evaluation plan for a program emerges from the philosophy and goals, as do all the other elements of the curriculum. Evaluation is a coconstituted process, one in which a value is given to changing patterns in light of a desired goal. Data collected in the comprehensive evaluation are interpreted, ordered, and used for decision making about the program. Methods used to obtain evaluation data are generally considered to be threefold; they are observation, interview, and survey. There are five major elements to an evaluation system: input, output, process, supplemental, and financial (Wolf, 1979).

Input refers to program precondition. Information gathered before entrance into the program establishes a baseline and includes data from the program pretest and from student profiles. The purpose of a program pretest is to ascertain the basic knowledge level of the students before they actually begin the program. When these data are later compared with posttest data, they demonstrate a dimension of what students have learned in the program. The profile includes information about student characteristics. The significant characteristics among these are age, gender, race, ethnic origin, marital status, educational background, significant work experience, Graduate Record Examination scores, scholarships and other academic honors, present work situation, nature of work, hours worked per week, academic references, professional references, and student status.

Output refers to program outcome. Data are collected at varying specified points during the educational process, at the end of each course, at the end of each level, and at the end of the program. Information is gathered at the end of each course from the following sources: 1) student self-evaluation and faculty evaluation of student performance, and 2) student and faculty evaluation of the overall conduct and effect of the course. Data gathered at the end of each level and at the end of the program denote student progress according to the goals and indicators. Faculty, independently and collectively, reflect on the performance of each student at each level and at the program's end, and arrive at a decision on the performance by each student on each level indicator. These data are compared with pretest data to determine student progress and the effectiveness of the program.

Process refers to program execution. Data are collected in this instance to determine whether or not the various types of learning opportunities described in the program plan are being implemented in a satisfactory manner. The data are obtained from three different sources: 1) observation through class visitation; 2) inspection of course documents, student papers, bibliographies, student projects, and other related and ancillary materials; and 3) faculty and student evaluations about the course process.

Supplemental refers to program effect. Data are gathered from program faculty and students, families for whom the students provided service, and the program graduates and their immediate supervisors in their place of employment. These data provide valuable information relative to perceptions of, reactions to, and opinions of the program among peer professionals in nursing and the community at large.

Financial, obviously, refers to program cost. The purpose of financial assessment is to determine the relative cost efficiency of the program. Data are collected in categories of both direct and indirect expenditures. Direct expenditures are instructional costs and program support costs. Indirect expenditures are instructional support costs and are sometimes difficult to identify clearly. Both direct and indirect expenditures are divided into basic and additional costs as well as into recurring and nonrecurring costs. The program financial evaluation plan, then, yields data on basic recurring costs, basic nonrecurring costs, additional recurring costs, and additional nonrecurring costs. The total amount of all costs is examined and evaluated in relation to the number of students in the program. Cost per student is then determined. The basic and additional recurring costs are used to project future costs of the program.

These five enumerated elements—input, output, process, supplemental, and financial—provide a clearly defined structure for a thorough and comprehensive assessment of a total program.

A Sample Curriculum Plan Consistent With the Human Becoming School of Thought

Many different curricular patterns may be designed with human becoming as the nursing theoretical base. Important in developing a curriculum plan, whatever its theoretical base, is that it has internal consistency. This means that the fundamental assumptions about the human-universe health process are consistent and recognized throughout the plan. Following is a sample curriculum plan consistent with the human becoming school of thought for a program leading to the master's of science degree in nursing. The sample plan includes purpose, philosophy, conceptual framework, themes, program goals and indicators, course plan, course sequence, and some instructional and evaluation strategies. It would be necessary to have a detailed program evaluation plan as well (see Parse, 1981).

Purpose of the Program

The purpose of the graduate program leading to a master of science degree in nursing is to provide a curriculum plan for guiding the learner in the achievement of certain goals that will

TABLE 5.3 Unifying Concepts, Support Theories, and Theorists

Program focus	Family health, leadership, inquiry
Nursing theoretical base	Human becoming
Nurse theorist	Parse
Unifying concepts	Meaning, rhythmicity, transcendence
Themes	Leading-following, teaching-learning, change-persistence, family process, interrogating-coming to know

Support Theories	Theorists
Change theory	J. H. van den Berg
	P. Watzlawick
Teaching-learning theory	J. Dewey
	M. Greene
	C. Rogers
Leadership theory	R. Burns
	P. Drucker
	T. Peters
Family theory	W. Kempler
Research theory	H.-G. Gadamer
	A. Giorgi
	A. Kaplan
	F. Kerlinger
	P. Ricoeur
	H. Spiegelberg
	A. van Kaam

broaden the theoretical knowledge base of the learner in prepa-ration for a leadership role and doctoral study. The nurse pre-pared at the master's level develops, tests, and evaluates con-cepts relevant to nursing and critically examines concepts and theories in relation to health issues, initiates nursing research, and practices nursing in a leadership role.

This master's program provides experience in the area of family health and in two specific areas of role concentration: teaching nursing and administering nursing services. All stu-dents will be provided the opportunity to learn the theoretical base of human becoming and, consistent with this opportunity, will participate in practicum experiences with specially selected families. Students selecting teaching nursing as their area of role concentration will be provided with the opportunity to learn the theoretical base of the teaching-learning process from the perspective of human becoming. Practicum experiences will be provided. Students selecting administering of nursing services as their area of role concentration will be provided with the opportunity to learn the theoretical base of the administrative process from the perspective of human becoming. Practicum experiences for these students will be situated in various health care settings. The teacher of nursing who successfully completes this program will have a specialization in family health and will be prepared to assume a junior faculty position. The administrator of nursing services who graduates from this program will be prepared to administer in a management position in a health care system.

Philosophy of the Program

The faculty believes that nursing is a scientific discipline, the practice of which is a performing art. Nurses provide leadership in service to society through a concern for families' health care and quality of living, and through participating in change. The phenomenon of concern to nursing is the human-universe-health process. The human becoming school of thought is the focus of nursing in this graduate program; thus, the unifying nursing framework encompasses the assumptions, principles, and methodologies. From a human becoming perspective, the human is an open being freely choosing meaning in situation, and health is becoming in mutual process with the universe. Nursing practice focuses on offering true presence to families in choosing possibilities in their changing health process. The nurse initiates nurse-person and nurse-group processes with families as they illuminate meaning, synchronize rhythms, and mobilize transcendence. The nurse regularly conducts self-evaluations and plans for continuing learning. Through human becoming research studies, the nurse enhances the evolution of the discipline. The Parse research method and the human becoming hermeneutic method are used to study lived experiences of health. Teacher and learner coconstitute the educational process through sharing knowledge and planning educationally sound and fulfilling experiences. Ideas are investigated regularly and systematically in an effort to discover new knowledge.

The graduate nursing program in this school of nursing prepares a human becoming family health nurse with an area of concentration in either teaching nursing or administering nursing services. The graduate nursing program emphasizes and concentrates on concept development, that is, the creating and testing of concepts. Also highlighted are theoretical foundations of leadership and rigorous methods of research. The program is directed mainly toward the evolution of nursing knowledge as a guide for practice, research, and education.

Conceptual Framework of the Program

The conceptual framework emerges quite naturally from the philosophy. The unifying concepts of the framework are meaning, rhythmicity, and transcendence, and the themes are leading-following, teaching-learning, change-persistence, family process, and interrogating-coming to know. Table 5.3 shows the unifying concepts, themes, support theories, and theorists.

Program Goals and Indicators

In this program, students and faculty coconstitute the teaching-learning process. Students are encouraged throughout to plan their own learning opportunities. Each student, with the assistance of faculty members, is expected to identify personal goals consistent with the program goals, plan experiences, and evaluate the achievement of goals. Program evaluation is a continuous process shared between and among students, faculty, and consumers. The program goals and indicators are as follows.

Goal 1: To practice nursing guided by the theory of human becoming.
  Indicators:

- Understands concepts related to human becoming.
- Lives the dimensions of the human becoming practice methodology with families.
- Initiates plans for personal change.
- Demonstrates accountability to families.
- Initiates collaborative relationships with families and other professionals.

Goal 2: To practice a leadership role of teaching nursing or administering nursing services from the theoretical base consistent with human becoming.
  Indicators:

- Promotes the delivery of quality health care through teaching nursing or administering nursing services.
- Promotes change in social systems consistent with the theoretical perspective of human becoming.
- Teaches nursing or administers nursing services consistent with the theoretical base of human becoming.
- Compares value priorities in decision making.
- Demonstrates accountability.

Goal 3: To use the process of inquiry.
  Indicators:

- Uses literature to support conclusions.
- Comprehends the ontological-methodological links in research.
- Conducts a formal research study on a lived experience.

Goal 4: To contribute to theory evolution in nursing.
  Indicators:

- Elaborates concepts from the perspective of human becoming.

- Develops unique concepts arising from the theory of human becoming.

Level Indicators for the Program

Two levels are identified in this graduate nursing program. Level 1 evaluation occurs after completion of the first 24 credits, and Level 2 evaluation after completion of 48 total credits in the program. Student progress is evaluated at Levels 1 and 2 in accordance with specific indicators.

Course Plan

The focus of the courses in this curriculum design is on advanced knowledge and the practice of the art of nursing science. The courses evolve from the level indicators, which evolve from the program indicators. The course design has three structural components: focal courses, subsidiary courses, and role courses.

Focal courses. Five 3-credit courses provide an opportunity for in-depth study: nursing as a discipline, concept development and theory evolution, inquiry, leadership, and family. All these courses are didactic. The focal courses in the curriculum with their module titles follow.

- *Nursing Science: Human Becoming:* Assumptions about the human and health; principles, concepts, and theoretical structures of human becoming
- *Concept Development and Theory Evolution:* The construction of the theory of human becoming; extant theories and theory evolution
- *Nursing Research 1:* Experimental research designs; descriptive research designs
- *Leadership Foundations:* Change and learning; change and decision making; change and evaluation

- *Family:* Family process, issues, contextual grounding, and themes

Subsidiary courses. A series of six 3-credit courses provides in-depth study of leadership, inquiry, and concept development in the family-nurse process. Five of these courses have nursing practice components and are didactic with a practicum. The didactic dimension of these courses provides learning opportunities in three areas: inquiry, concept development, and leadership. The practicum dimension of these courses provides learning opportunities in using concepts as guides to nurse-family process. Practicum time is spent with families, in individual consultation with faculty, and in peer review seminars. One of these courses is an independent research project that provides learning opportunities in expanding concepts through a pilot study. The subsidiary courses in this curriculum, with their module titles, follow.

- *Nurse-Family Process 1:* Family health; meaning and health possibilities
- *Nurse-Family Process 2:* Evolutionary and planned change; persistence in change
- *Nurse-Family Process 3:* Health myths and metaphors; multicultural transformations
- *Family Patterns of Relating:* Struggle and commitment in nurse-family process; cocreating becoming
- *Family Life Experiences:* Meaning and family life experiences; transformations
- *Nursing Research 2:* Independent research project

Role courses. There are five 3-credit courses in the role concentration areas of teaching nursing and administering nursing services. These courses provide an opportunity for in-depth study in inquiry, leadership, and concept enhancement. Two of these five courses are required courses in each of the role areas. Of these two, one in each area is didactic and the other has both didactic and practicum components. The didactic courses provide opportunities related to the learning process in the teaching role area and related to the administrative process in the administering of nursing services role area. The courses with both a didactic and a practicum dimension provide opportunities to study and use concepts as guides in a leadership role. These courses and module titles follow.

Teaching Nursing Role Area:
- *Curriculum Process:* curriculum development process; curriculum plan
- *Teaching Nursing Practicum:* Teaching nursing model; ethical responsibilities inherent in being a teacher of nursing

Administering Nursing Role Area:
- *Administrative Process:* structure of administrative process; administrative plan
- *Administering Nursing Practicum:* Administering nursing services model; ethical responsibilities inherent in being a nurse administrator

Electives:
Three of the five role courses are electives. These courses are didactic and provide an opportunity for students to choose three of five possible options. The electives embellish aspects of the role areas and encourage in-depth study in the topics offered. The five elective options in the curriculum, with their module titles, follow.

- *Political Issues in Nursing Leadership:* Participation in health policy making; legal-ethical-moral responsibilities in nursing leadership roles
- *Nursing Leadership and Technological Resources:* Science and technology; use of technological resources in leadership situations
- *Comparative Studies in Nursing Leadership:* Education and administration in the People's Republic of China; education and administration in Europe
- *Nursing Leadership and Health Care Systems:* Peer professional relationships; change strategies in a multicultural system

- *Nursing Leadership and Institutions of Higher Learning:* Academic disciplines; change strategies in academia

Course Sequence

The graduate program leading to a master of science degree in nursing may be obtained through completion of a 48-credit curriculum plan. This program may be completed on a full- or part-time basis.

Instructional Strategies

Some instructional strategies used in this graduate nursing program are faculty-student process, nurse-family process, student-student process, teacher-student process, administrator-nurse process, and student-group process.

Faculty-student process is the interrelationship that evolves between teacher and student. Faculty and student collaborate from initial curriculum planning throughout the educational experience. Faculty guide students in one-to-one relationships and in small groups in each course in the graduate nursing program.

Nurse-family process is an evolving engagement of a family with the nursing student. In each subsidiary course, students live the human becoming theory as a guide to practice in the nurse-family process. Students are in true presence with families while living the dimensions and processes of the human becoming practice methodology. Supervising and evaluating are accomplished through review of video recordings of the nurse-family processes. These recordings are analyzed by students and faculty for the purpose of student supervision and evaluation. The videotape, as a mechanism supporting this instructional strategy, offers the student an opportunity to view the nurse-family process to identify concepts for further development.

Student-student process emerges among students as they develop peer professional relationships. Peer collaboration and evaluation are encouraged through small-group projects and peer review sessions related to nurse-family process, teacher-student process, and administrator-nurse process. Students share the opportunity to interrogate and enhance concepts in the process of concept development, inquiry, and leadership. All subsidiary and role courses use student-student process as an instructional strategy.

Teacher-student process is an instructional strategy for all students in the teaching role area. Each student teacher of nursing creates a teaching model that is used in a teaching situation. Use of the model entails teaching-learning opportunities with students of nursing. Interrelationships between the student teacher of nursing and nursing students are videotaped for analysis, supervision, and evaluation.

Administrator-nurse process is an instructional strategy for all students participating in the administering of nursing services role area. The student administrator of nursing services creates an administration model that is used in a health care setting. Use of the model entails working with staff nurses and other health care providers. Interrelationships between the student administrator of nursing services and the staff nurses and health care providers are videotaped for analysis, supervision, and evaluation.

Student-group process is an instructional strategy that encourages the student to develop skills in planning and organizing goals with others. It further offers students the opportunity to guide group process. Some student-group process sessions are videotaped for analysis, supervision, and evaluation. Student-group process is used in all courses.

Evaluation Strategies

Evaluation strategies consistent with the human becoming perspective are particular to the courses, but, in general, the evaluations in all courses include quality of performance in group process, written and oral examinations, performance in nurse-family process, and quality of written assignments and oral presentations.

CODA

The human becoming school of thought presented in this book provides a foundation from which new questions can be raised about phenomena of concern to nursing and other health care disciplines. This school of thought will continue to evolve through creative conceptualization and research. The knowledge gained will guide further research and practice and offer a challenge to nurse educators to implement nursing programs consistent with this human science paradigmatic perspective. The 1981 edition of this book set forth a path to journey on the cutting edge of the discipline of nursing. The journey has been filled with intense and quiet moments, pleasures and challenges all-at-once. It continues to be one of forging new cutting-edge paths and living with opportunities that arise with the emergence of the ever new mysteries of the yet-to-be discovered possibilities in sciencing and living the art of human becoming for the betterment of humankind.

GLOSSARY

All-at-once: Mutual processing

Coconstitution: Coparticipation in creating meaning in situation

Cocreate: Coconstitute

Coexistence: Living with predecessors, contemporaries, and successors all-at-once

Concept: Idea; one's conceptualization of a precept

Connecting-separating: Being with and apart from others, ideas, objects, and situations all-at-once

Cotranscending: Moving with

Enabling-limiting: Living the opportunities-restrictions present in all choosings all-at-once

Facticity: The givens in a situation arising from prior choosings

Historicity: One's becoming over time

Imaging: Reflective-prereflective coming to know the explicit-tacit all-at-once

Intentionality: A tenet specifying that the human is a deliberate being-present-with the world

Intersubjectivity: Subject-to-subject true presence

Languaging: Signifying valued images through speaking-being silent and moving-being still

Meta metaperspective: One's view of the other's view of the view

Metaperspective: One's view of the other's view

Not-yet: Multidimensional possibilities not known explicitly

Originating: Inventing new ways of conforming-not conforming in the certainty-uncertainty of living

Paradigm: Ontological view of a particular field of study; a worldview

Paradox: Unity of apparent opposites; two dimensions of one rhythm

Paradoxical: An apparent contradiction

Pattern: A configuration of the human-universe process

Patterns of relating: Paradoxical ways of becoming

Perspectival view: One angle of a phenomenon

Phenomenology: The study of phenomena as they appear

Possibles: The imaginables

Powering: The pushing-resisting process of affirming-not affirming being in light of nonbeing

Prereflective choosing: Tacitly making a decision without explicit consideration

Principle: A professed rule of action

Project: A human creation

Reflective choosing: Explicitly considering options in decision making

Revealing-concealing: Disclosing-not disclosing all-at-once

Rhythmical: Cadent

Situated freedom: Unencumbered option to choose in each situation

Subjectivity: Inherent unitary human nature

Tenet: A basic belief

Theoretical structure: A nondirectional statement interrelating concepts

Transcending: Moving with; exceeding

Transforming: Shifting the view of the familiar-unfamiliar; the changing of change in coconstituting anew in a deliberate way

True presence: Genuine, nonmechanical, nonroutinized attentiveness to the other(s)

Unitary: Different from the sum of parts

Valuing: Confirming-not confirming cherished beliefs in light of a personal worldview

REFERENCES

Bandler, R., & Grinder, J. (1975a). *Patterns of the hypnotic techniques of Milton H. Erickson* (Vol. I). Cupertino, CA: Meta.

Bandler, R., & Grinder, J. (1975b). *The structure of magic I.* Palo Alto, CA: Science & Behavior Books.

Banonis, B. C. (1989). The lived experience of recovering from addiction: A phenomenological study. *Nursing Science Quarterly, 2,* 37-43.

Baumann, S. L. (1994). No place of their own: An exploratory study. *Nursing Science Quarterly, 7,* 162-169.

Bruteau, B. (1979). *The psychic grid: How we create the world we know.* Wheaton, IL: Theosophical Publishing House.

Buber, M. (1965). *The knowledge of man* (M. Friedman, Ed.). New York: Harper & Row.

Bunkers, S. S. (in press). Considering tomorrow: Parse's theory-guided research. *Nursing Science Quarterly.*

Chopra, D. (1989). *Quantum healing.* New York: Bantam.

Chopra, D. (1993). *Ageless body; timeless mind.* New York: Harmony.

Cody, W. K. (1991). Grieving a personal loss. *Nursing Science Quarterly, 4,* 61-68.

Cody, W. K. (1994). Meaning and mystery in nursing science and art. *Nursing Science Quarterly, 7,* 48-51.

Cody, W. K. (1995a). The lived experience of grieving, for families living with AIDS. In R. R. Parse (Ed.), *Illuminations: The human becoming theory in practice and research* (pp. 197-142). New York: National League for Nursing Press.

Cody, W. K. (1995b). Of life immense in passion, pulse, and power: Dialoguing with Whitman and Parse—A hermeneutic study. In R. R. Parse (Ed.), *Illuminations: The human becoming theory in practice and research* (pp. 269-307). New York: National League for Nursing Press.

Costello-Nickitas, D. M. (1994). Choosing life goals: A phenomenological study. *Nursing Science Quarterly, 7*, 87-92.

Cousins, N. (1983). *The healing heart.* New York: Norton.

Cousins, N. (1989). *Head first: The biology of hope.* New York: E. D. Dutton.

Dacher, E. (1997). Healing values: What matters in healthcare. *Noetic Sciences Review, 42*, 10-15, 49-51.

Daly, J. (1995).The lived experience of suffering. In R. R. Parse (Ed.), *Illuminations: The human becoming theory in practice and research* (pp. 243-268). New York: National League for Nursing Press.

Davis, D. K., & Cannava, E. (1995). The meaning of retirement for communally-living retired performing artists. *Nursing Science Quarterly, 8*, 8-16.

Dilthey, W. (1961). *Pattern and meaning in history: Thoughts on history and society* (H. P. Rickman, Ed. & Trans.). New York: Harper & Row.

Dilthey, W. (1976). *Selected writings* (H. P. Rickman, Trans.). Cambridge, UK: Cambridge University Press.

Dilthey, W. (1977a). Ideas concerning a descriptive and analytic psychology. In R. M. Zaner & K. L. Heiges (Trans.), *Descriptive psychology and historical understanding* (pp. 23-120). The Hague: Martinus Nijhoff. (Original work published 1894)

Dilthey, W. (1977b). The understanding of other persons and their expressions of life. In R. M. Zaner & K. L. Heiges (Trans.), *Descriptive psychology and historical understanding* (pp. 123-144). The Hague: Martinus Nijhoff. (Original work published 1927)

Dilthey, W. (1988). *Introduction to the human sciences* (R. J. Betanzos, Trans.). Detroit: Wayne State University Press. (Original work published 1883)

Dossey, L. (1982). *Space, time and medicine.* Boulder, CO: Shambhala.

Dossey, L. (1984). *Beyond illness: Discovering the experience of health.* Boulder, CO: Shambhala.

Dossey, L. (1991). *Meaning and medicine: A doctor's tales of breakthrough and healing.* New York: Bantam.

Dossey, L. (1993). *Healing words: The power of prayer and the practice of medicine.* San Francisco: Harper.

Dubos, R. (1979a). Human ecology. In D. S. Sobel (Ed.), *Ways of health: Holistic approaches to ancient and contemporary medicine* (pp. 387-396). New York: Harcourt Brace Jovanovich.

Dubos, R. (1979b). Medicine evolving. In D. S. Sobel (Ed.), *Ways of health: Holistic approaches to ancient and contemporary medicine* (pp. 21-44). New York: Harcourt Brace Jovanovich.

Ellis, R. (1977). Fallabilities, fragments, and frames: Contemplations of research in medical-surgical nursing. *Nursing Research, 26*(3), 181.

Ermarth, M. (1978). *Wilhelm Dilthey: The critique of historical reason.* Chicago: University of Chicago Press.

Ferguson, M. (1980). *The Aquarian conspiracy: Personal and social transformation in the 1980s.* Los Angeles: Tarcher.

Frankl, V. E. (1959). *The will to meaning.* New York: New American Library.

Frankl, V. E. (1967). Significance of the meaning of health. In D. R. Belgium (Ed.), *Religion and medicine: Essays on meaning, valuing, and health* (pp. 177-185). Ames: Iowa State University Press.

Futrell, M., Wondolowski, C., & Mitchell, G. J. (1993). Aging in the oldest old living in Scotland: A phenomenological study. *Nursing Science Quarterly, 6,* 189-194.

Gadamer, H.-G. (1975). *Truth and method* (G. Graden & J. Cumming, Eds. & Trans.). New York: Seabury.

Gadamer, H.-G. (1976). *Philosophical hermeneutics* (D. E. Linge, Trans.). Berkeley: University of California Press.

Gadamer, H.-G. (1993). *Truth and method* (2nd rev. ed.) (Translation revised by J. Weinsheimer & D. G. Marshall). New York: Continuum.

Giorgi, A. (1970). *Psychology as a human science.* New York: Harper & Row.

Giorgi, A. (1971). Phenomenology and experimental psychology: II. In A. Giorgi, W. Fischer, & R. von Eckartsberg (Eds.), *Duquesne studies in phenomenological psychology* (Vol. 1, pp. 3-29). Pittsburgh, PA: Duquesne University Press.

Giorgi, A. (1985). Sketch of a psychological phenomenological method. In A. Giorgi (Ed.), *Phenomenology and psychological research* (pp. 8-22). Pittsburgh, PA: Duquesne University Press.

Goldstein, K. (1959). Health as value. In A. H. Maslow (Ed.), *New knowledge in human values* (p. 87). Chicago: Henry Regnery.

Gouty, C. A. (1996). *Feeling alone while with others.* Unpublished doctoral dissertation, Loyola University, Chicago.

Greene, M. (1978). *Landscapes of learning.* New York: Teachers College Press.

Grinder, J., & Bandler, R. (1976). *The structure of magic II.* Palo Alto, CA: Science & Behavior Books.

Hall, B. P. (1976). *The development of consciousness: A confluent theory of values.* New York: Paulist.

Hall, E. T. (1976). *Beyond culture.* Garden City, NY: Doubleday/Anchor.

Harman, W. (1997). Biology revisioned. *Noetic Sciences Review, 41,* 12-17, 39-42.

Heidegger, M. (1962). *Being and time* (J. Macquarrie & E. Robinson, Trans.). New York: Harper & Row.

Jonas, C. M. (1992). The meaning of being an elder in Nepal. *Nursing Science Quarterly, 5,* 171-175.

Jonas, C. M. (1995). Evaluation of the human becoming theory in family practice. In R. R. Parse (Ed.), *Illuminations: The human becoming theory in practice and research* (pp. 347-366). New York: National League for Nursing Press.

Jourard, S. M. (1971). *The transparent self.* New York: Van Nostrand Reinhold.

Kelley, L. S. (1991). Struggling with going along when you do not believe. *Nursing Science Quarterly, 4,* 123-129.

Kempler, W. (1974). *Principles of gestalt family therapy.* Costa Mesa, CA: Kempler Institute.

King, I. M. (1981). *A theory for nursing: Systems, concepts, process.* Albany, NY: Delmar.

King, S. (1981). *Imagineering for health.* Wheaton, IL: Theosophical Publishing House.

Kuhn, T. S. (1970). *The structure of scientific revolutions.* Chicago: University of Chicago Press.

Laing, R. D., Phillipson, H., & Lee, A. R. (1966). *Interpersonal perception: A theory and a method of research.* New York: Harper & Row.

Langer, S. (1976). *Philosophy in a new key.* Cambridge, MA: Harvard University Press.

Leininger, M. (1996). Culture care theory, research, and practice. *Nursing Science Quarterly, 9,* 71-80.

Leonard, G. (1978). *The silent pulse.* New York: E. D. Dutton.

LeShan, L. (1982). *The mechanic and the gardener.* New York: Holt, Rinehart & Winston.

Liberman, J. (1991). *Light: Medicine of the future.* Santa Fe: Bear.

Macquarrie, J. (1968). *Martin Heidegger.* Richmond, VA: John Knox.

Mann, J. (1997). Medicine and public health, ethics and human rights. *The Hastings Center Report, 27*(3), 6-13.

Marcel, G. (1978). *Mystery of being: Reflection and mystery* (Vol. 1). South Bend, IN: Gateway Editions.

Merleau-Ponty, M. (1963). *The structure of behavior.* Boston: Beacon.

Merleau-Ponty, M. (1973). *The prose of the world.* Evanston, IL: Northwestern University Press.

Merleau-Ponty, M. (1974). *Phenomenology of perception* (C. Smith, Trans.). New York: Humanities Press.

Mitchell, G. J. (1990). The lived experience of taking life day-by-day in later life: Research guided by Parse's emergent method. *Nursing Science Quarterly, 3,* 29-36.

Mitchell, G. J. (1993). Living paradox in Parse's theory. *Nursing Science Quarterly, 6,* 44-51.

Mitchell, G. J. (1994). The meaning of being a senior: Phenomenological research and interpretation with Parse's theory of nursing. *Nursing Science Quarterly, 7,* 70-79.

Mitchell, G. J. (1995). Evaluation of the human becoming theory in practice in an acute care setting. In R. R. Parse (Ed.), *Illuminations: The human becoming theory in practice and research* (pp. 367- 399). New York: National League for Nursing Press.

Moyers, B. (1993). *Healing and the mind.* Garden City, NY: Doubleday.

Neuman, B. (1982). *The Neuman systems model: Application to nursing education and practice.* Norwalk, CT: Appleton-Century-Crofts.

Newman, M. A. (1979). *Theory development in nursing.* Philadelphia: Davis.

Newman, M. A. (1994). *Health as expanding consciousness.* New York: National League for Nursing Press.

Nietzsche, F. (1968). *The will to power* (W. Kaufmann, Ed. & Trans.). New York: Vintage.

Nightingale, F. (1946). *Notes on nursing: What it is and what it is not.* Philadelphia: J. B. Lippincott. (First edition printed in 1859)

Nokes, K. M., & Carver, K. (1991). The meaning of living with AIDS: A study using Parse's theory of man-living-health. *Nursing Science Quarterly, 4,* 175-179.

Northrup, D. T., & Cody, W. K. (in press). Evaluation of the human becoming theory in practice in an acute care psychiatric setting. *Nursing Science Quarterly.*

Orem, D. E. (1995). *Nursing: Concepts of practice.* St. Louis, MO: C. V. Mosby-Year Book.

Parse, R. R. (1981). *Man-living-health: A theory of nursing.* New York: John Wiley.

Parse, R. R. (1987). *Nursing science: Major paradigms, theories, and critiques.* Philadelphia: W. B. Saunders.

Parse, R. R. (1989). Parse's man-living-health model and administration of nursing service. In B. Henry, C. Arndt, M. DiVincenti, & A. Marriner-Tomey (Eds.), *Dimensions of nursing administration: Theory, research, education, practice* (pp. 69-74). Boston: Blackwell Scientific.

Parse, R. R. (1990a). Health: A personal commitment. *Nursing Science Quarterly, 3,* 136-140.

Parse, R. R. (1990b). Parse's research methodology with an illustration of the lived experience of hope. *Nursing Science Quarterly, 3,* 9-17.

Parse, R. R. (1992). Human becoming: Parse's theory of nursing. *Nursing Science Quarterly, 5,* 35-42.

Parse, R. R. (1993). The experience of laughter: A phenomenological study. *Nursing Science Quarterly, 6,* 39-43.

Parse, R. R. (1994a). Charley Potatoes or mashed potatoes? *Nursing Science Quarterly, 7,* 97.

Parse, R. R. (1994b). Laughing and health: A study using Parse's research method. *Nursing Science Quarterly, 7,* 55-64.

Parse, R. R. (1994c). Quality of life: Sciencing and living the art of human becoming. *Nursing Science Quarterly, 7,* 16-21.

Parse, R. R. (Ed.). (1995). *Illuminations: The human becoming theory in practice and research.* New York: National League for Nursing Press.

Parse, R. R. (1996a). Building knowledge through qualitative research: The road less traveled. *Nursing Science Quarterly, 9,* 10-17.

Parse, R. R. (1996b). Quality of life for persons living with Alzheimer's disease: The human becoming perspective. *Nursing Science Quarterly, 9.* 126-133.

Parse, R. R. (1996c). Reality: A seamless symphony of becoming. *Nursing Science Quarterly, 9,* 181-184.

Parse, R. R. (1997a). The human becoming theory: The was, is, and will be. *Nursing Science Quarterly, 10,* 32-38.

Parse, R. R. (1997b). Joy-sorrow: A study using the Parse research method. *Nursing Science Quarterly, 10,* 80-87.

Parse, R. R. (1997c). The language of nursing knowledge: Saying what we mean. In I. M. King & J. Fawcett (Eds.), *The language of nursing theory and metatheory* (pp. 73-77). Indianapolis: Center Nursing Press.

Parse, R. R., Coyne, A. B., & Smith, M. J. (1985). *Nursing research: Qualitative methods.* Bowie, MD: Brady.

Paterson, J., & Zderad, L. T. (1976). *Humanistic nursing.* New York: John Wiley.

Peplau, H. E. (1952). *Interpersonal relations in nursing.* New York: Putnam.

Petardi, L. A. (in press). Weathering the storm: Persevering through a difficult time. *Nursing Science Quarterly.*

Pilkington, F. B. (1993). The lived experience of grieving the loss of an important other. *Nursing Science Quarterly, 6,* 130-139.

Polanyi, M. (1958). *Personal knowledge.* Chicago: University of Chicago Press.

Polanyi, M. (1959). *The study of man.* Chicago: University of Chicago Press.

Polanyi, M. (1969). *Knowing and being.* Chicago: University of Chicago Press.

Polkinghorne, D. E. (1983). *Methodology for the human sciences: Systems of inquiry.* Albany: State University of New York Press.

Raths, L. E., Harmin, M., & Simon, S. B. (1978). *Values and teaching: Working with values in the classroom.* Columbus, OH: Merrill.

Rendon, D. C., Sales, R., Leal, I., & Piqué, J. (1995). The lived experience of aging in community-dwelling elders in Valencia, Spain: A phenomenological study. *Nursing Science Quarterly, 8,* 152-157.

Ricoeur, P. (1974). *The conflict of interpretations: Essays in hermeneutics* (W. Domingo et al., Trans.). Evanston, IL: Northwestern University Press.

Ricoeur, P. (1984). *Time and narrative, Vol. 1* (K. McLaughlin & D. Pellauer, Trans.). Chicago: University of Chicago Press.

Ricoeur, P. (1985). *Time and narrative, Vol. 2* (K. McLaughlin & D. Pellauer, Trans.). Chicago: University of Chicago Press.

Ricoeur, P. (1987). *The rule of metaphor: Multidisciplinary studies of the creation of meaning in language* (R. Czerny et al., Trans.). Toronto: University of Toronto Press.

Ricoeur, P. (1988). *Time and narrative, Vol. 3* (K. Blamey & D. Pellauer, Trans.). Chicago: University of Chicago Press.

Ricoeur, P. (1992). *History and truth* (C. A. Kelbley, Trans.). Evanston, IL: Northwestern University Press.

Rogers, M. E. (1970). *An introduction to the theoretical basis of nursing.* Philadelphia: Davis.

Rogers, M. E. (1986). Science of unitary human beings. In V. Malinski (Ed.), *Explorations on Martha Rogers' science of unitary human beings* (pp. 3-8). Norwalk, CT: Appleton-Century-Crofts.

Rogers, M. E. (1990). Nursing: Science of unitary irreducible human beings: Update 1990. In E. A. M. Barrett (Ed.), *Visions of Rogers' science-based nursing* (pp. 5-11). New York: National League for Nursing Press.

Rogers, M. E. (1992). Nursing science and the space age. *Nursing Science Quarterly, 5,* 27-34.

Roy, C., & Andrews, H. A. (1991). *The Roy adaptation model: The definitive statement.* E. Norwalk, CT: Appleton & Lange.

Santopinto, M. D. A., & Smith, M. C. (1995). Evaluation of the human becoming theory in practice with adults and children. In R. R. Parse (Ed.), *Illuminations: The human becoming theory in practice and research.* New York: National League for Nursing Press.

Sapir, E. (1966). *Culture, language and personality.* Berkeley: University of California Press.

Sartre, J.-P. (1966). *Being and nothingness.* New York: Washington Square.

Schutz, A. (1967). On multiple realities. In M. Natanson (Ed.), *The problem of social reality: Collected papers* (Vol. 1, pp. 209-212). The Hague: Martinus Nijhoff.

Shakespeare, W. (1978). Hamlet (II, II, 218). In A. L. Rowse (Ed.), *The annotated Shakespeare.* New York: Clarkson N. Potter. (Original work published 1600)

Siegel, B. S. (1989). *Peace, love and healing.* New York: Harper & Row.

Smith, M. C. (1990). Struggling through a difficult time for unemployed persons. *Nursing Science Quarterly, 3,* 18-28.

Sontag, S. (1979). *Illness as metaphor.* New York: Vintage.

Spiegelberg, H. (1976). *The phenomenological movement* (Vols. 1, 2). The Hague: Martinus Nijhoff.

Straus, E. W. (1974). Sounds, words, sentences. In E. W. Straus (Ed.), *Language and language disturbances* (pp. 81-105). New York: Humanities Press.

Thornburg, P. D. (1993). *The meaning of hope in parents whose infants died from sudden death syndrome.* Doctoral dissertation, University of Cincinnati. (University Microfilms International No. 9329939)

Tillich, P. (1952). *The courage to be.* New Haven, CT: Yale University Press.

Tillich, P. (1954). *Love, power and justice.* New York: Oxford University Press.

Toben, B. (1975). *Space-time and beyond.* New York: E. P. Dutton.

van den Berg, J. H. (1971). Phenomenology and metabletics. *Humanitas, 7*(3), 285.

van Kaam, A. (1974). Existential crisis and human development. *Humanitas, 10*(2), 109-126.

van Kaam, A., van Croonenburg, B., & Muto, S. (1969). *The participant self* (Vol. 2). Pittsburgh, PA: Duquesne University Press.

von Bertalanffy, L. (1959). Human values in a changing world. In A. H. Maslow (Ed.), *New knowledge in human values.* New York: Harper.

Wang, C. E. (1997). *Mending a torn fish net: A metaphor for hope.* Unpublished doctoral dissertation, Loyola University, Chicago.

Watson, J. (1988). New dimensions of human caring theory. *Nursing Science Quarterly, 1,* 175-181.

Watzlawick, P. (1978). *The language of change.* New York: Basic Books.

Watzlawick, P., Weakland, J., & Fisch, R. (1974). *Change: Principles of problem formation and problem resolution.* New York: Norton.

Weil, A. (1995). *Spontaneous healing.* New York: Knopf.

Weisskopf, W. A. (1959). Existence and values. In A. H. Maslow (Ed.), *New knowledge in human values*. New York: Harper.

White, L. A. (1938). Science is sciencing. *Philosophy of Science, 5*(4), 369-389.

Whorf, B. E. (1956). *Language, thought and reality*. Cambridge: Technology.

Wolf, R. (1979). *Evaluation in education*. New York: Praeger.

Wondolowski, C., & Davis, D. K. (1991). The lived experience of health in the oldest old: A phenomenological study. *Nursing Science Quarterly, 4,* 113-118.

BIBLIOGRAPHY

Abbott, E. A. (1952). *Flatland.* New York: Dover.

Adler, C. S., Stanford, G., & Morrissey, S. (Eds.). (1976). *We are but a moment's sunlight.* New York: Simon & Schuster.

Alinsky, S. D. (1969). *Reveille for radicals.* New York: Random House.

Alinsky, S. D. (1972). *Rule for radicals.* New York: Random House.

Anderson. R. T. (1972). *Anthropology: A perspective on man.* Belmont, CA: Wadsworth.

Andrus, K. (1995). Parse's nursing theory and the practice of perioperative nursing. *Canadian Operating Room Nursing Journal, 13*(3), 19-22.

Arndt, M. J. (1995). Parse's theory of human becoming in practice with hospitalized adolescents. *Nursing Science Quarterly, 8,* 86-90.

Ballard, E. G. (1978). *Man and technology.* Atlantic Highlands, NJ: Humanities Press.

Bannon, J. F. (1967). *The philosophy of Merleau-Ponty.* New York: Harcourt, Brace, and World.

Banonis, B. C. (1995). Metaphors in the practice of the human becoming theory. In R. R. Parse (Ed.), *Illuminations: The human becoming theory in practice and research* (pp. 87-95). New York: National League for Nursing Press.

Barnett, L. (1948). *The universe and Dr. Einstein.* New York: Bantam.

Barrett, W. (1965). *What is existentialism?* New York: Grove.

Beauchamp, C. (1990). *The lived experience of struggling with making a decision in a critical life situation.* Unpublished doctoral dissertation, University of Miami, FL.

Belgium, D. R. (Ed.). (1967). *Religion and medicine: Essays of meaning, valuing and health.* Ames: Iowa State University Press.

Benhabib, S. (1992). *Situating the self: Gender, community, and postmodernism in contemporary ethics*. New York: Routledge.

Bentov, I. (1977). *Stalking the wild pendulum*. New York: E. P. Dutton.

Berger, P. L., & Luckmann, T. (1966). *The social construction of reality*. Garden City, NY: Doubleday.

Berry, E. E. (1992). *Curved thought and textual wandering: Gertrude Stein's postmodernism*. Ann Arbor: University of Michigan Press.

Besant, A. (1903). *Thought power: Its control and culture*. Wheaton, IL: Theosophical Publishing House.

Birkerts, S. (1994). *The Gutenberg elegies: The fate of reading*. New York: Faber & Faber.

Birringer, J. H. (1991). *Theater, theory, postmodernism*. Bloomington: Indiana University Press.

Blanchard, D. (1996). *Intimacy as a lived experience of health*. Unpublished doctoral dissertation, Wayne State University, Detroit.

Bok, S. (1978). *Lying: Moral choice in public and private life*. New York: Pantheon.

Bolen, J. S. (1979). *The Tao of psychology: Synchronicity and the self*. San Francisco: Harper & Row.

Born, M. (1962). *Einstein's theory of relativity* (rev. ed). New York: Dover.

Briggs, J. (1988). *Fire in the crucible: The alchemy of creative genius*. New York: St. Martin's.

Briggs, J., & Peat, F. (1989). *Turbulent mirror*. New York: Harper & Row.

Briggs, J. P., & Peat, F. (1984). *Looking glass universe: The emerging science of wholeness*. New York: Simon & Schuster.

Brooker, P. (Ed.). (1992). *Modernism/postmodernism*. New York: Longman.

Bruner, J. (1990). *Acts of meaning*. Cambridge, MA: Harvard University Press.

Bruner, J. S. (1960). *The process of education*. New York: Random House.

Buber, M. (1970). *I and thou*. New York: Schribner.

Busch, T. W., & Gallagher, S. (Eds.). (1992). *Merleau-Ponty, hermeneutics, and postmodernism*. Albany: State University of New York Press.

Butler, M. J. (1988). Family transformation: Parse's theory in practice. *Nursing Science Quarterly, 1*, 68-74.

Butler, M. J., & Snodgrass, F. G. (1991). Beyond abuse: Parse's theory in practice. *Nursing Science Quarterly, 4*, 76-82.

Buytendyk, F. J. J. (1974). *Prolegomena to an anthropological physiology*. Atlantic Highlands, NJ: Humanities Press.

Calder, N. (1979). *Einstein's universe*. New York: Viking.

Callinicos, A. (1990). *Against postmodernism: A Marxist critique*. New York: St. Martin's.

Campbell, J. (1973). *The hero with a thousand faces*. Princeton, NJ: Princeton University Press.

Camus, A. (1946). *The stranger*. New York: Random House.

Camus, A. (1995). *The first man* (D. Hapgood, Trans.). New York: Knopf.

Capra, F. (1976). *The Tao of physics*. New York: Bantam.

Carroll, L. (1960). *The annotated Alice: Alice's adventures in wonderland;* and *Through the looking glass.* Cleveland: World.

Castaneda, C. (1972). *Journey to Ixtlan: The lessons of Don Juan.* New York: Simon & Schuster.

Castaneda, C. (1974). *Tales of power.* New York: Simon & Schuster.

Castaneda, C. (1977). *The second ring of power.* New York: Simon & Schuster.

Caughie, P. L. (1991). *Virginia Woolf and postmodernism: Literature in quest and question of itself.* Urbana: University of Illinois Press.

Cheetham, M. A. (1991). *Remembering postmodernism: Trends in recent Canadian art.* Toronto: Oxford University Press.

Cody, W. K. (1995). The meaning of grieving for families living with AIDS. *Nursing Science Quarterly, 8,* 104-114.

Cody, W. K. (1995). True presence with families living with HIV disease. In R. R. Parse (Ed.), *Illuminations: The human becoming theory in practice and research* (pp. 115-133). New York: National League for Nursing Press.

Cody, W. K., Hudepohl, J. H., & Brinkman, K. S. (1995). True presence with a child and his family. In R. R. Parse (Ed.), *Illuminations: The human becoming theory in practice and research* (pp. 135- 146). New York: National League for Nursing Press.

Cody, W. K., & Mitchell, G. J. (1992). Parse's theory as a model for practice: The cutting edge. *Advances in Nursing Science, 15*(2), 52-65.

Colaizzi, P. F. (1978). *Technology and dwelling: The secrets of life and death.* Unknown: Author.

Collingwood, R. D. (1956). *The idea of history.* New York: Oxford University Press.

Connor, S. (1989). *Postmodernist culture: An introduction to theories of the contemporary.* New York: Basil Blackwell.

Crichton, M. (1991). *Jurassic Park.* New York: Ballantine.

Crowther, P. (1993). *Critical aesthetics and postmodernism.* New York: Oxford University Press.

Csikszentmihalyi, M. (1996). *Creativity: Flow and the psychology of discovery and invention.* New York: HarperCollins.

Daly, J., Mitchell, G. J., & Jonas-Simpson, C. M. (1996). Quality of life and the human becoming theory: Exploring discipline-specific contributions. *Nursing Science Quarterly, 9,* 170-174.

Darwin, C. (1979). *Origin of species.* New York: Hill and Wang.

Day, C. (1990). *Places of the soul: Architecture and environmental design as a healing art.* Northamptonshire, UK: Aquarian.

de Beauvoir, S. (1948). *The ethics of ambiguity.* Secaucus. NJ: Citadel.

de Beauvoir, S. (1977). *A very easy death.* New York: Warner.

de Bono, E. (1967). *New think.* New York: Hearst.

de Chardin, T. (1965). *The phenomenon of man.* New York: Harper & Row.

de Chardin, T. (1966). *On love and suffering.* New York: Paulist.

Derrida, J. (1976). *On grammatology.* Baltimore, MD: Johns Hopkins University Press.

Derrida, J. (1991). *A Derrida reader: Between the blinds* (P. Kamuf, Ed.). New York: Columbia University Press.

Dewey, J. (1922). *Human nature and conduct.* New York: Modern Library.

Dilthey, W. (1976). *Selected writings* (H. P. Rickman, Trans.). Cambridge, UK: Cambridge University Press.

Dilthey, W. (1988). *Introduction to the human sciences* (R. J. Betanzos, Trans.). Detroit: Wayne State University Press. (Original work published 1883)

Docherty, T. (1990). *After theory: Postmodernism/postmarxism.* New York: Routledge.

Docherty, T. (Ed.). (1993). *Postmodernism: A reader.* New York: Columbia University Press.

Doherty, J., Graham, E., & Malek, M. (Eds.). (1992). *Postmodernism and the social sciences.* New York: St. Martin's.

Doll, W. (1993). *A post-modern perspective on curriculum.* New York: Teachers College Press.

Drucker, P. (1992). *Managing the future: The 1990s and beyond.* New York: NAL/Dutton.

Dubin, R. (1969). *Theory building.* New York: Free Press.

Dubos, R. (1970). *Man adapting.* New Haven, CT: Yale University Press.

Einstein, A. (1946). *The meaning of relativity.* Princeton, NJ: Princeton University Press.

Englehardt, H. T., Jr., & Callahan, D. (Eds.). (1977). *Knowledge, value and belief* (Vol. 2). New York: The Hastings Center, Institute of Society, Ethics and the Life Sciences.

Evans-Wenty, W. Y. (1978). *The Tibetan book of the dead.* London: Oxford University Press.

Feifel, H. (Ed.). (1965). *The meaning of death.* New York: McGraw-Hill.

Feyerabend, P. (1988). *Against method.* New York: Verso.

Feyerabend, P. (1991). *Three dialogues on knowledge.* Cambridge, MA: Basil Blackwell.

Fischer, C. T., & Brodsky, S. L. (Eds.). (1978). *Client participation in human services: The Prometheus principle.* New Brunswick, NJ: Transaction.

Fisher, A. L. (1969). *The essential writings of Merleau-Ponty.* New York: Harcourt, Brace, and World.

Fletcher, J. (1975). *Situation ethics.* Philadelphia: Westminster.

Foucault, M. (1970). *The order of things: An archaeology of the human sciences.* New York: Vintage.

Foucault, M. (1973). *The birth of the clinic.* London: Tavistock.

Foucault, M. (1980). *Power knowledge. Selected interviews and other writings 1927-1977* (C. Gordon, Ed.). Brighton, UK: Harvester.

Frankl, V. E. (1960). *The doctor and the soul.* New York: Knopf.

Frankl, V. E. (1972). *Man's search for meaning.* New York: Simon & Schuster.

Frazier, C. A. (1974). *Faith healing: Finger of God? or scientific curiosity?* New York: Thomas Nelson.

Frazier, K. (Ed.). (1991). *The hundredth monkey and other paradigms of the paranormal.* Buffalo, NY: Prometheus.

Freire, P. (1989). *Pedagogy of the oppressed.* New York: Continuum.

Fromm, E. (1963). *The art of loving.* New York: Harper & Row.

Fromm, E. (1968). *The revolution of hope.* New York: Harper & Row.

Gary, W., Duhl, F. J., & Rizzo, N. D. (Eds.). (1969). *General systems theory and psychiatry.* Boston: Little, Brown.

Gates, B. (1995). *The road ahead.* New York: Viking Penguin.

Gaylin, W. (1979). *Feelings.* New York: Harper & Row.

Ghiselin, B. (Ed.). (1952). *The creative process.* Berkeley: University of California Press.

Giorgi, A., Knowles, R., & Smith, D. L. (Eds.). (1979). *Phenomenological psychology* (Vol. 2). Pittsburgh, PA: Duquesne University Press.

Gleick, J. (1987). *Chaos: Making a new science.* New York: Penguin.

Goffman, E. (1959). *The presentation of self in everyday life.* Garden City, NY: Doubleday/ Anchor.

Goffman, E. (1961). *Asylums.* New York: Doubleday/Anchor.

Goffman, E. (1967). *Interactional ritual: Essays on face-to-face behavior.* Garden City, NY: Doubleday/Anchor.

Goffman, E. (1974). *Frame analysis.* New York: Harper & Row.

Goldberg, P. (1983). *The intuitive edge: Understanding and developing intuition.* Los Angeles: Tarcher.

Gordon, D. (1978). *Therapeutic metaphors.* Cupertino, CA: Meta.

Guba, E., & Lincoln, Y. (1989). *Fourth generation evaluation.* Newbury Park, CA: Sage.

Habermas, J. (1968). *Knowledge and human interests.* Boston: Beacon.

Hageman, L. (1977). *In the midst of winter.* Denville, NJ: Dimension.

Hall, B. A., & Parse, R. R. (1993). The theory-research-practice triad. Commentary: The inherent value of practice theories. Response: Theory guides research and practice. *Nursing Science Quarterly, 6,* 10-12.

Hawking, S. W. (1988). *A brief history of time: From the big bang to black holes.* New York: Bantam.

Heidegger, M. (1972). *On time and being* (J. Stambaugh, Trans.). New York: Harper & Row.

Heine, C. (1991). Development of gerontological nursing theory: Applying the man-living-health theory of nursing. *Nursing and Health Care, 12*(4), 184-188.

Hempel, C. G. (1966). *Philosophy of natural science.* Englewood Cliffs, NJ: Prentice Hall.

Husserl, E. (1965). *Phenomenology and the crisis of philosophy.* Philadelphia: Harper & Row.

Jacobs, J. (1961). *The death and life of great American cities.* New York: Vintage.

Jacono, B. J., & Jacono, J. J. (1994). Holism: The teacher is the method. *Nurse Education Today, 14*(4), 287-291.

Jacono, B. J., & Jacono, J. J. (1996). The benefits of Newman and Parse in helping nurse teachers determine methods to enhance student creativity. *Nurse Education Today, 16*(5), 356-362.

Jasper, D. (Ed.). (1992). *Postmodernism, literature and the future of theology.* New York: St. Martin's.

Jencks, C. (1991). *The language of postmodern architecture* (6th ed.). London: Academy.

Johnston, C. M. (1986). *The creative imperative: A four-dimensional theory of human growth and planetary evolution.* Berkeley, CA: Celestial Arts.

Jonas, C. M. (1994). True presence through music. *Nursing Science Quarterly, 7,* 102-103.

Jonas, C. M. (1995). True presence through music for persons living their dying. In R. R. Parse (Ed.), *Illuminations: The human becoming theory in practice and research* (pp. 97-104). New York: National League for Nursing Press.

Jonas-Simpson, C. (1996). The patient-focused care journey: Where patients and families guide the way. *Nursing Science Quarterly, 9,* 145-146.

Josselson, R. (1992). *The space between us: Exploring the dimensions of human relationships.* San Francisco: Jossey-Bass.

Kaplan, A. (1961). *The new world of philosophy.* New York: Random House.

Kaplan, A. (1964). *The conduct of inquiry: Methodology for behavioral sciences.* Scranton, PA: Chandler.

Keen, S. (1960). *Apology for wonder.* New York: Harper & Row.

Keen, S. (1967). *Gabriel Marcel.* Richmond, VA: John Knox.

Keen, S. (1970). *To a dancing God.* New York: Harper & Row.

Keleman, S. (1975). *Living your dying.* New York: Random House.

Kelley, L. S. (1995). Parse's theory in practice with a group in the community. *Nursing Science Quarterly, 8,* 127-132.

Kessey, K. (1962). *One flew over the cuckoo's nest.* New York: Viking.

Kikuchi, J., & Simmons, H. (Eds.). (1992). *Philosophic inquiry in nursing.* Newbury Park, CA: Sage.

Klotz, H. (1988). *The history of postmodern architecture.* Cambridge: MIT Press.

Kockelmans, J. J. (Ed.). (1967). *Phenomenology.* Garden City, NY: Doubleday.

Koelb, C. (Ed.). (1990). *Nietzsche as postmodernist: Essays pro and contra.* Albany: State University of New York Press.

Koestler, A. (1974). *Janus: A summing up.* New York: Vintage.

Kraft, W. F. (1974). *A psychology of nothingness.* Philadelphia: Westminster.

Kruse, B. (in press). The lived experience of serenity: Using Parse's research method. *Nursing Science Quarterly.*

Kuhns, W. (1969). *Environmental man.* New York: Harper & Row.

Kundera, M. (1988). *The art of the novel* (L. Asher, Trans.). New York: Grove. (Original work published 1986)

Kung, H. (1988). *Theology for a third millennium.* Garden City, NY: Doubleday.

Kurtz, P. (1977). *Exuberance: A philosophy of happiness.* Buffalo, NY: Prometheus.

Laing, R. D. (1970). *The divided self.* Baltimore, MD: Pelican.

Laing, R. D. (1970). *The politics of experience.* New York: Ballantine.

Laing, R. D. (1972). *The politics of the family.* New York: Random House.

Lamont, C. (1977). *The philosophy of humanism.* New York: Frederick Ungar.

Langer, S. K. (1980). *Philosophy in a new key: A study in the symbolism of reason, rite, and art.* Cambridge, MA: Harvard University Press.

Lanham, R. A. (1993). *The electronic word: Democracy, technology, and the arts.* Chicago: University of Chicago Press.

Laswell, H. (1958). *Politics: Who gets what, when, how.* New York: World.

Laswell, H. (1976). *Power and personality.* New York: Norton.

Lather, P. (1991). *Getting smart: Feminist research and pedagogy within the postmodern.* New York: Routledge.

Laudan, L. (1978). *Progress and its problems.* Berkeley: University of California Press.

Leininger, M. (1978). *Transcultural nursing: Concepts, theories and practices.* New York: John Wiley.

Lemkow, A. F. (1990). *The wholeness principle.* Wheaton, IL: Quest.

Leonard, G. (1972). *The transformation.* New York: Dell.

LeShan, L. (1977). *You can fight for your life.* New York: M. Evans.

Lieber, L. R., & Lieber, H. G. (1936). *The Einstein theory of relativity.* New York: Rinehart.

Liehr, P. R. (1989). The core of true presence: A loving center. *Nursing Science Quarterly, 2,* 7-8.

Lightman, A. (1993). *Einstein's dream.* New York: Pantheon.

Lui, S. L. (1993). *The meaning of health in hospitalized older women in Taiwan.* Doctoral dissertation, University of Colorado Health Sciences Center, Denver.

Lujipen, W. A. (1960). *Existential phenomenology.* New York: Humanities Press.

Mann, F. (1972). *Acupuncture.* New York: Random House.

Marcel, G. (1956). *The philosophy of existentialism.* Secaucus, NJ: Citadel.

Marcel, G. (1964). *Creative fidelity.* New York: Noonday.

Martin, M. L., Forchuk, C., Santopinto, M., & Butcher, H. K. (1992). Alternative approaches to nursing practice: Application of Peplau, Rogers, and Parse. *Nursing Science Quarterly, 5,* 80-85.

Maslow, A. H. (1968). *Toward a psychology of being.* Princeton, NJ: Van Nostrand.

Maslow, A. H. (Ed.). (1971). *New knowledge in human values.* Chicago: Henry Regnery.

Maslow, A. H. (1973). *The farther reaches of human nature.* New York: Viking.

Mason, H. (1970). *Gilgamesh: A verse narrative.* Boston: New American Library.

Mattice, M. (1991). Parse's theory of nursing in practice: A manager's perspective. *Canadian Journal of Nursing Administration, 4*(1), 11-13.

Mattice, M., & Mitchell, G. J. (1990). Caring for confused elders. *The Canadian Nurse, 86*(11), 16-18.

Mavely, R., & Mitchell, G. J. (1994). Consider karaoke: An audiovisual device that encourages client participation with music. *Canadian Nurse, 90,* 22-24.

May, R. (1967). *Man's search for himself.* New York: Norton.

May, R. (1972). *Power and innocence: A search for the sources of violence.* New York: Norton.

May, R. (1975). *The courage to create.* Toronto: George J. McLeod.

Mayeroff, M. (1971). *On caring.* New York: Harper & Row.

McClelland, D. C. (1975). *Power: The inner experience.* New York: Irvington.

McGowan, J. (1991). *Postmodernism and its critics.* Ithaca, NY: Cornell University Press.

McHale, B. (1992). *Constructing postmodernism.* New York: Routledge.

McLuhan, M., & Fiore, Q. (1967). *The medium is the message.* New York: Bantam.

Melnechenko, K. L. (1995). Parse's theory of human becoming: An alternative guide to nursing practice for pediatric oncology nurses (with commentary by R. R. Parse). *Journal of Pediatric Oncology Nursing, 12*(3), 122-128.

Mendelsohn, R. S. (1979). *Confessions of a medical heretic.* Chicago: Contemporary.

Mendoza, R. G. (1995). *The acentric labyrinth.* Rockport, MA: Element.

Mitchell, G. J. (1986). Utilizing Parse's theory of man-living-health in Mrs. M's neighborhood. *Perspectives, 10*(4), 5-7.

Mitchell, G. J. (1988). Man-living-health: The theory in practice. *Nursing Science Quarterly, 1,* 120-127.

Mitchell, G. J. (1990). Struggling in change: From the traditional approach to Parse's theory-based practice. *Nursing Science Quarterly, 3,* 170-176.

Mitchell, G. J. (1991). Nursing diagnosis: An ethical analysis. *Image: Journal of Nursing Scholarship, 23*(2), 99-103.

Mitchell, G. J. (1993). Parse's theory in practice. In M. E. Parker (Ed.), *Patterns of nursing theories in practice* (pp. 62-80). New York: National League for Nursing Press.

Mitchell, G. J. (1993). Time and a waning moon: Seniors describe the meaning to later life. *The Canadian Journal of Nursing Research, 25*(1), 51-66.

Mitchell, G. J. (1995). The lived experience of restriction-freedom in later life. In R. R. Parse (Ed.), *Illuminations: The human becoming theory in practice and research* (pp. 159-195). New York: National League for Nursing Press.

Mitchell, G. J. (1996). Pretending: A way to get through the day. *Nursing Science Quarterly, 9,* 92-93.

Mitchell, G. J. (1996). A reflective moment with false cheerfulness. *Nursing Science Quarterly, 9,* 53-54.

Mitchell, G. J., & Copplestone, C. (1990). Applying Parse's theory to perioperative nursing: A nontraditional approach. *AORN Journal, 51*(3), 787-798.

Mitchell, G. J., & Heidt, P. (1994). The lived experience of wanting to help another. *Nursing Science Quarterly, 7,* 119-127.

Mitchell, G. J., & Pilkington, B. (1990). Theoretical approaches in nursing practice: A comparison of Roy and Parse. *Nursing Science Quarterly, 3,* 81-87.

Mitchell, G. J., & Santopinto, M. D. A. (1988). An alternative to nursing diagnosis. *The Canadian Nurse, 84*(1), 25-28.

Montagu, A. (1972). *Touching.* New York: Harper & Row.

Montagu, A., & Matson, F. (1979). *The human connection*. New York: McGraw-Hill.

Moustakas, C. E. (1961). *Loneliness*. Englewood Cliffs, NJ: Prentice Hall.

Moustakas, C. E. (1972). *Loneliness and love*. Englewood Cliffs, NJ: Prentice Hall.

Moustakas, C. E. (1974). *The self*. New York: Harper & Row.

Moustakas, C. E. (1975). *The touch of loneliness*. Englewood Cliffs, NJ: Prentice Hall.

Moustakas, C. E. (1977). *Creative life*. New York: Van Nostrand Reinhold.

Moustakas, C. E. (1990). *Heuristic research*. Newbury Park, CA: Sage.

Naisbitt, J. (1994). *Global paradox*. New York: William Morrow.

Naisbitt, J., & Aburdene, P. (1990). *Megatrends 2000: Ten new directions*. New York: William Morrow.

Natanson, M. (Ed.). (1967). *The problem of social reality. Collected papers, Vol. 1*. The Hague: Martinus Nijhoff.

Newman, M. (1994). *Health as expanding consciousness* (2nd ed.). New York: National League for Nursing Press.

Newton, I. (1974). *The mathematical papers of Isaac Newton* (Vol. 6) (D. Whiteside, Ed.). Cambridge, UK: Cambridge University Press. (Original works published 1684-1691)

Nicholson, L. J. (Ed.). (1990). *Feminism/postmodernism*. New York: Routledge.

Nicolis, G., & Prigogine, I. (1989). *Exploring complexity*. New York: Freeman.

Nierenberg, G. I., & Calero, H. (1973). *Meta-talk: The guide to hidden meanings in conversation*. New York: Simon & Schuster.

Nietzsche, F. (1973). *Thus spoke Zarathustra*. New York: Viking.

Noddings, N. (1984). *Caring: A feminine approach to ethics and moral development*. Berkeley: University of California Press.

Norris, C. (1990). *What's wrong with postmodernism: Critical theory and the ends of philosophy*. Baltimore, MD: Johns Hopkins University Press.

Norris, C. (1992). *Uncritical theory: Postmodernism, intellectuals and the Gulf War*. Amherst: University of Massachusetts Press.

Norris, C. (1993). *The truth about postmodernism*. Cambridge, MA: Basil Blackwell.

Northrup, D. (1995). *Exploring the experience of time passing for persons with HIV disease: Parse's theory-guided research*. Doctoral dissertation, University of Austin, TX. (University Microfilms International No. 9534912)

Ogilvy, J. (1977). *Many dimensional man*. New York: Harper & Row.

Olsen, L. (1990). *Circus of the mind in motion: Postmodernism and the comic vision*. Detroit: Wayne State University Press.

Ornstein, R. E. (1969). *On the experience of time*. New York: Penguin.

Ornstein, R. E. (1972). *The psychology of consciousness*. San Francisco: Freeman.

Orr, L. (Ed.). (1991). *Yeats and postmodernism* (1st ed.). Syracuse, NY: Syracuse University Press.

Parse, R. R. (1993). Parse's human becoming theory: Its research and practice implications. In M. E. Parker (Ed.), *Patterns of nursing theories in practice* (pp. 49-61). New York: National League for Nursing Press.

Parse, R. R. (1996). The human becoming theory: Challenges in practice and research. *Nursing Science Quarterly, 9,* 55-60.

Perkins, R. L. (1976). *Søren Kierkegaard.* Atlanta: John Knox.

Perloff, M. (1990). *Poetic license: Essay on modernist and postmodernist lyric.* Evanston, IL: Northwestern University Press.

Perls, F. S. (1969). *Gestalt therapy verbatim.* Lafayette, CA: Real People.

Peter, L. J., & Hull, R. (1970). *The Peter principle.* New York: Bantam.

Phillips, D. C. (1976). *Holistic thought in social science.* Stanford, CA: Stanford University Press.

Pilkington, B. (1997). *Persisting while wanting to change: Research guided by Parse's theory.* Unpublished doctoral dissertation, Loyola University, Chicago.

Pirsig, R. M. (1980). *Zen and the art of motorcycle maintenance.* New York: Bantam.

Polanyi, M. (1966). *The tacit dimension.* Garden City, NY: Doubleday/Anchor.

Popper, K. R., Sir. (1959). *The logic of scientific discovery.* New York: Basic.

Prather, H. (1970). *Notes to myself.* Moab, UT: Real People.

Prather, H. (1972). *I touch the earth, the earth touches me.* Garden City, NY: Doubleday.

Prather, H. (1977). *Notes on love and courage.* Garden City, NY: Doubleday.

Prigogine, I., & Stengers, I. (1984). *Order out of chaos: Man's new dialogue with nature.* Boulder, CO: Shambhala.

Quiquero, A., Knights, D., & Meo, C. O. (1991). Theory as a guide to practice: Staff nurses choose Parse's theory. *Canadian Journal of Nursing Administration,* 4(1), 14-16.

Rasmusson, D. L. (1995). True presence with homeless persons. In R. R. Parse (Ed.), *Illuminations: The human becoming theory in practice and research* (pp. 105-113). New York: National League for Nursing Press.

Rasmusson, D. L., Jonas, C. M., & Mitchell, G. J. (1991). The eye of the beholder: Applying Parse's theory with homeless individuals. *Clinical Nurse Specialist,* 5(3), 139-143.

Redfield, J. (1993). *The celestine prophesy.* New York: Warner.

Redfield, J. (1996). *The tenth insight.* New York: Warner.

Ricoeur, P. (1981). *Hermeneutics and the human-sciences* (J. B. Thompson, Trans.). Paris: Cambridge.

Ricoeur, P. (1992). *Oneself as another* (K. Blamey, Trans.). Chicago: University of Chicago Press.

Riehl, J. P., & Roy, C. (1980). *Conceptual models for nursing practice.* New York: Appleton-Century-Crofts.

Rilke, R. M. (1964). *The notebooks of Malte Laurids Brigge.* New York: Norton.

Roberts, J. (1990). *Postmodernism, politics and art.* Manchester, UK: Manchester University Press.

Rogers, C. E., & Stevens, B. (1971). *Person to person: The problem of being human.* New York: Pocket Books.

Rogers, M. E. (1961). *Educational revolution in nursing.* New York: Macmillan.

Rosenthal, T. (1973). *How could I not be among you.* New York: George Braziller.

Rucker, R. (1984). *The fourth dimension: A guided tour of the higher universes.* Boston: Houghton Mifflin.

Sacks, O. (1989). *Seeing voices.* Los Angeles: University of California Press.

Sacks, O. C. (1995). *An anthropologist on Mars.* New York: Knopf.

Sallis, J. (1973). *Phenomenology and the return to beginnings.* New York: Humanities Press.

Santopinto, M. D. A. (1989). The relentless drive to be ever thinner: A study using the phenomenological method. *Nursing Science Quarterly, 2,* 29-36.

Sartre, J.-P. (1963). *Search for a method.* New York: Knopf.

Sartre, J.-P. (1964). *Nausea.* New York: New Dimensions.

Sartre, J.-P., & Levy, B. (1996). *Hope now: The 1980 interviews* (A. van den Hoven, Trans.). Chicago: University of Chicago Press.

Sarup, M. (1988). *Post-structuralism and postmodernism.* New York: Harvester Wheatsheaf.

Sarup, M. (1993). *An introductory guide to post structuralism and post modernism.* Athens: University of Georgia Press.

Sayers, D. L. (1971). *Are women human?* Grand Rapids, MI: William B. Eerdmans.

Schon, D. (1983). *The reflective practitioner.* New York: Basic.

Schumacher, E. F. (1973). *Small is beautiful.* New York: Harper & Row.

Schutz, A. (1975). *On phenomenology and social relations.* Chicago: University of Chicago Press.

Schutz, W. C. (1967). *Joy.* New York: Grove.

Selye, H. (1950). *The stress of life.* New York: McGraw-Hill.

Shostrom, E. L. (1968). *Man the manipulator.* New York: Bantam.

Silverman, H. J. (Ed.). (1990). *Postmodernism: Philosophy and arts.* New York: Routledge.

Sim, S. (1992). *Beyond aesthetics: Confrontations with poststructuralism and postmodernism.* Toronto: University of Toronto Press.

Skinner, Q. (Ed.). (1990). *The return of grand theory in the human sciences.* Cambridge, MA: Cambridge University Press.

Smith, H. (1982). *Beyond the post-modern mind.* Wheaton, IL: Theosophical Publishing House.

Smith, M. C. (1990). Pattern in nursing practice. *Nursing Science Quarterly, 3,* 57-59.

Smith, R. G. (1975). *Martin Buber.* Atlanta, GA: John Knox.

Smith, T. (1992). *Dialectical social theory and its critics: From Hegel to analytical Marxism and postmodernism.* Albany: State University of New York Press.

Smyth, E. J. (Ed.). (1991). *Postmodernism and contemporary fiction.* London: Batsford.

Sobel, D. S. (Ed.). (1979). *Ways of health: Holistic approaches to ancient and contemporary medicine.* New York: Harcourt Brace Jovanovich.

Spenceley, S. M. (1995). The CNS in multidisciplinary pulmonary rehabilitation: A nursing science perspective. *Clinical Nurse Specialist, 9*(4), 192-198.

Spiegelberg, H. (1976). *The phenomenological movement* (Vols. 1 and 2). The Hague: Martinus Nijhoff.

Stevens, W. (1942). *The necessary angel*. New York: Random House.

Strasser, S. (1963). *Phenomenology and the human sciences*. Pittsburgh, PA: Duquesne University Press.

Strasser, S. (1969). *The idea of dialogal phenomenology*. Pittsburgh, PA: Duquesne University Press.

Styles, M., & Moccia, P. (1993). *On nursing: A literary celebration*. New York: National League for Nursing Press.

Swimme, B., & Berry, T. (1993). *The universe story: From the primordial flaring forth to the Ecozdic era*. San Francisco: Harper.

Szasz, T. S. (1974). *The myth of mental illness* (rev. ed.). New York: Harper & Row.

Tarnas, R. (1993). *The passion of the Western mind*. New York: Ballantine.

Tillich, P. (1955). *The new being*. New York: Scribner.

Tillich, P. (1963). *The new eternal now*. New York: Scribner.

Toffler, A. (1970). *Future shock*. New York: Random House.

Toffler, A. (Ed.). (1974). *Learning for tomorrow: The role of the future in education*. New York: Random House.

Toulmin, S. (1960). *The philosophy of science*. New York: Harper & Row.

Toulmin, S. (1982). *The return to cosmology*. Berkeley: University of California Press.

Toulmin, S. (1990). *Cosmopolis. The agenda of modernity*. New York: Free Press.

Tournier, P. (1973). *The meaning of persons*. New York: Harper & Row.

Towers, B. (1975). *Teilhard de Chardin*. Atlanta, GA: John Knox.

Toynbee, A. (1976). *Mankind and mother earth*. New York: Oxford University Press.

van den Berg, J. H. (1966). *The psychology of the sick bed*. Pittsburgh, PA: Duquesne University Press.

van den Berg, J. H. (1970). *Things: Four metabletic reflections*. Pittsburgh, PA: Duquesne University Press.

van Kaam, A. (1966). *The art of existential counseling*. Wilkes-Barre, PA: Dimension.

van Kaam, A. (1969). *Existential foundations of psychology*. Garden City, NY: Doubleday.

van Kaam, A. (1970). *On being involved*. Denville, NJ: Dimension.

van Kaam, A. (1972). *Living creatively*. Denville, NJ: Dimension.

van Kaam, A. (1972). *On being yourself*. Denville, NJ: Dimension.

van Kaam, A. (Ed.). (1974). Conflict and change. *Humanitas, 10*(2).

van Kaam, A. (Ed.). (1975). Silence and saying: The expressive dimension of the self. *Humanitas, 11*(2).

van Kaam, A. (Ed.). (1979). The freedom of the human. *Humanitas, 15*(3).

van Kaam, A. (Ed.). (1979). The value of the human. *Humanitas, 15*(2).

van Kaam, A. (Ed.). (1980). Spirituality and originality. *Studies in Formative Spirituality, 1*(1).

van Kaam, A. (Ed.). (1980). Spirituality and the desert experience. *Studies in Formative Spirituality, 1*(2).

van Kaam, A., van Croonenburg, B., & Muto, S. (1968). *The emergent self.* Wilkes-Barre, PA: Dimension.

van Kaam, A., van Croonenburg, B., & Muto, S. (1969). *The participant self* (Vol. 1). Pittsburgh, PA: Duquesne University Press.

Van Perusen, C. (1972). *A phenomenology and reality.* Pittsburgh, PA: Duquesne University Press.

von Bertalanffy, L. (1968). *General system theory: Foundations, development, applications.* New York: George Braziller.

Waldrop, M. (1992). *Complexity.* New York: Simon & Schuster.

Walker, C. A. (1996). Coalescing the theories of two nurse visionaries: Parse and Watson. *Journal of Advanced Nursing, 24*(5), 988-996.

Watts, A. W. (1951). *The wisdom of insecurity.* New York: Pantheon.

Watzlawick, P. (1974). *An anthology of human communication, text and tape.* Palo Alto, CA: Science & Behavior Books.

Watzlawick, P. (1977). *How real is real?* New York: Vintage.

Watzlawick, P., Beavin, J., & Jackson, D. D. (1967). *Pragmatics of human communication: A study of interactional patterns, pathologies, and paradoxes.* New York: Norton.

Waugh, P. (Ed.). (1992). *Postmodernism: A reader.* New York: E. Arnold.

Wellmer, A. (1991). *The persistence of modernity: Essays on aesthetics, ethics and postmodernism.* Cambridge: MIT Press.

Wertenbaker, L. T. (1974). *Death of a man.* Boston: Beacon.

White, J., & Krippner, S. (Eds.). (1977). *Future science.* Garden City, NY: Doubleday.

Whitehead, A. (1978). *Process and reality* (Rev. ed; D. R. Griffin & D. W. Sherburne, Eds.). New York: Free Press. (Original work published 1929)

Whitehead, A. N. (1925). *Science and the modern world.* New York: Macmillan.

Whitehead, A. N. (1938). *Modes of thought.* New York: Free Press.

Whitehead, A. N. (1969). *Process and reality.* New York: Free Press.

Willman, A. (1996). *Health is living: A theoretical and empirical analysis of the concept of health with examples from geriatric nursing care.* Doctoral dissertation, Lunden University, Stockholm, Sweden.

Wimpenny, P. (1993). The paradox of Parse's theory. *Senior Nurse, 13*(5), 10-13.

Wolf, M. (1992). *A thrice told tale: Feminism, postmodernism, and ethnographic responsibility.* Stanford, CA: Stanford University Press.

Zaner, R., & Ihde, D. (1973). *Phenomenology and existentialism.* New York: Putnam.

Zurbrugg, N. (1993). *The parameters of postmodernism.* Carbondale, IL: Southern Illinois University Press.

INDEX

ABOUT THE AUTHOR

Rosemarie Rizzo Parse, RN, PhD, FAAN, is Professor and Niehoff Chair at Loyola University Chicago. She is founder and editor of *Nursing Science Quarterly*; president of Discovery International, Inc., which sponsors international nursing theory conferences; and founder of the Institute of Human Becoming, where she teaches the ontological, epistemological, and methodological aspects of the human becoming school of thought. Her most recent work is *Illuminations: The Human Becoming Theory in Practice and Research* (National League for Nursing Press, 1995). Previous works include *Nursing Fundamentals; Man-Living-Health: A Theory of Nursing; Nursing Science: Major Paradigms, Theories, and Critiques;* and *Nursing Research: Qualitative Methods* (coauthored). Her theory is a guide for practice in health care settings in the United States, Canada, Finland, and Sweden; her research methodology is used as a method of inquiry by nurse scholars in Australia, Canada, Denmark, Finland, Greece, Italy, Japan, South Korea, Sweden, the United Kingdom, and the United States. She is a graduate of Duquesne University in Pittsburgh and received her master's and doctorate from the University of Pittsburgh. She was on the faculty of the University of Pittsburgh; was dean of the Nursing School at Duquesne University; and, from 1983 to 1993, was professor and coordinator of the Center for Nursing Research at Hunter College of the City University of New York.

She also has been a visiting professor at the University of Cincinnati, the University of South Carolina, Wright State University, the University of Western Sydney (Australia), and Florida Atlantic University, where she was the first Christine E. Lynn Eminent Scholar in Nursing.